"Brian's compassion, wisdom, sens[...] new parents at ease come through o[...] advocate for new and working parents, I'm thrilled to see such a practical, honest guide to make sure new dads are as informed and engaged as possible, every step of the way."

—**Jessica Shortall**, author of *Work. Pump. Repeat*, and
TED speaker on the case for paid family leave

"Authored by one of the few male birth doulas in the US, this book is a one-of-a-kind resource for expectant dads and birth partners. Inclusive in tone, this gem of a book shares birth and breastfeeding advice that can be useful to ALL expectant parents regardless of their gender or sexual orientation. The relationship and emotional wellness pointers provided throughout give much-needed support and guidance on labor and breastfeeding support, postpartum depression, and much more! The perfect baby shower gift for any dad-to-be, this book is the *only* resource fathers will need to be fully engaged birth partners and parents."

—**Robbie Davis-Floyd, PhD**, author of *Birth as an
American Rite of Passage* and *Ways of Knowing about Birth*

"Have now read the book, and what can I say? Well, number one, wish I could say I wrote this. Often, I have felt dads were left on the sidelines either because they were passive or felt they were in the way. Of course, things have changed, and Brian has very succinctly described how partners can be both helpful and a participant in this most important experience in one's life—in order to build a healthy, lasting relationship for a family and marriage. I think this book is a must for all new parents-to-be. This should be an included part of every new OB packet. It will be for my patients."

—**Robert E. Schorlemer, MD, FACOG**, clinical practice
of obstetrics and gynecology

"It should be mandatory that every soon-to-be father has to read this. Brian made the biggest difference with my husband on our fourth child. My only regret is that I didn't know him sooner. I didn't know that the birthing process could be so easy, and for the first time ever, I didn't want to choke my husband in the delivery room! Brian changed my caveman into a caring partner that was so helpful and not annoying at all. Trust me, buy this for every man you know having a child soon, first born or not! It's a huge game changer."

—**Erica Rico**, morning show host,
KKBQ-FM 93Q Houston

"As a pediatrician, I hear from fathers almost daily that they don't feel they have a role in their growing child. Brian the Birth Guy empowers dads through knowledge of what to expect, focus on bolstering relationships, and problem-solving techniques to help manage dad's new responsibilities. Luckily, this guide is also really helpful for moms too!"

—**Sky Izaddoost, MD, FAAP**, pediatrician at
the Children's Hospital of San Antonio
Primary Care-Stone Oak

"If an expectant dad wants to be a champion in the delivery room, they should definitely read this book. It is the *only* comprehensive guide available in bookstores that covers all aspects of pregnancy, childbirth, and breastfeeding from a birth partner's point of view. Brian Salmon's many years of hands-on experience in the delivery and recovery room make him uniquely qualified to provide practical, time-tested pointers that you won't find anywhere else."

—**Stuart "Dr. Stu" Fischbein, OB-GYN**, founder of
Birthing Instincts, and coauthor of *Fearless Pregnancy*

"Finally! A book for dads-to-be! This is a must-read for any partner about to jump into the perilous birth journey to parenthood. Evidence-based as well as anecdotal, Brian and Kirsten cover everything from how to get your relationship ready for a rocky labor ride, your important role in this messy but exciting process, how to cope with the postpartum reverberation, and beyond. I have worked with Brian through numerous births and he tells it like it is—this is the real stuff! Read this book and become her hero!"

—**Kelly Morales, MD**, obstetrician and gynecologist

"This book should be read by every dad who truly desires to be a partner in this amazing journey of pregnancy."

—**David Ghozland, MD**, obstetrician and gynecologist

"This should be at the top of the baby shower list for any soon-to-be dad! I love Brian's passion for equipping dads in this wild journey called "Fatherhood." This book is loaded with useful information for those of us who want to be the best partner for our spouse and absolutely rock it as a dad!"

—**Adam Busby**, Star of TLC's *Outdaughtered*, and
father to quintuplets

"Finally, dads have their own *What to Expect*-style guide made just for them. From pregnancy, labor and delivery, and navigating the first few months with baby, Brian's guide is fun and easy to read. Best, it helps dads feel empowered and included in the entire process, even nursing!"

—**Rachel Pitzel, Esq**, content creator and social media
influencer @xo.rachelpitzel

THE BIRTH GUY'S
GO-TO GUIDE
FOR
NEW
DADS

How to Support Your Partner Through
Birth, Breastfeeding & Beyond

Brian W. Salmon,
DAD, DOULA & CERTIFIED LACTATION COUNSELOR

Kirsten Brunner, MA, LPC

New Harbinger Publications, Inc.

Distributed in Canada by Raincoast Books

Copyright © 2019 by Brian W. Salmon and Kirsten Brunner
        New Harbinger Publications, Inc.
        5674 Shattuck Avenue
        Oakland, CA 94609
        www.newharbinger.com

JEDI and related trademarks incorporating the word JEDI are registered trademarks of Lucasfilm Entertainment Company Ltd. LLC and are used in this book pursuant to the Fair Use Doctrine. No sponsorship or endorsement by, and no affiliation with, the trademark owner are claimed or implied by the author or publisher.

Cover design by Amy Shoup

Interior design by Michele Waters-Kermes

Acquired by Jess O'Brien

Edited by James Lainsbury

Illustrations by Isabel Hillock Davidson

Library of Congress Cataloging-in-Publication Data on file

21   20   19

10   9   8   7   6   5   4   3   2   1   First Printing

This book is dedicated to the many phenomenal dads and birth partners we've worked with through the years. You inspire and motivate us daily with your commitment to your families and your enthusiasm for the birth adventure.

—Brian and Kirsten

Contents

Foreword

A little over eighteen years ago, I began the journey into fatherhood when my oldest was born a mere five pounds and fifteen ounces. I remember when our son entered this world like it was yesterday. A fierce shrill cry exited his lungs as the doctor assisted him into our universe, and my heart melted the moment he was placed in my arms. While this moment, forever emblazoned in my mind, was joyful, I was scared as hell about what was to come.

No one can fully prepare you for the new role you are about to experience as a dad. But there is one guy who can get you pretty close.

I first met Brian when he called my office more than four years ago. He was insistent about connecting with me to share his story of being a dad and a doula. I agreed to meet one day in LA over lunch and found that we had a lot in common. We are both dads, and we both have a mission to empower men to take on their new role of fatherhood with confidence. I had been building my company, Diaper Dude, for over fifteen years when we first met. Since then, his passion and commitment to fatherhood has continued to impress me. He has once again outdone himself with this guide to assist dads on their journey into fatherhood.

As you take on this new role, I encourage you to be open, honest, and patient. Brian can help you achieve that with this book. He lays out everything you need to know about your partner and how you can make her feel secure as she prepares to deliver your newborn. Keep in mind that there are moments when we all fail, but it is from this failure that we learn to be better parents.

Today the role of dad is changing dramatically. Embrace this change and get involved with parenting. With Brian's help, you are sure to succeed.

—Chris Pegula
Creator of the company Diaper Dude and
award-winning author of *From Dude to Dad:
The Diaper Dude Guide to Pregnancy.*

Introduction

If you are reading this book, I believe some congratulations are in order. Congrats on beginning a journey toward parenthood! Double congrats on wanting to take an active role in the experience. That puts you in an emerging group of twenty-first-century dads and birth partners who are not content to sit on the sidelines. You *want* to help your partner through the pregnancy and birth. You're ready to take an active role in feeding, soothing, and caring for your baby. You are a modern-day parent, and you're looking for the information and advice needed to be a fully involved partner. This book is going to give you all of the tools and advice needed to do just that.

I was in your shoes more than thirteen years ago, when I was waiting for my first daughter to be born. The birth was an incredible, life-changing experience, but, to be perfectly honest, I didn't feel as prepared as I thought I should be. There simply weren't enough resources or classes directed at dads. Sure, there were some books and workshops for parents, but they didn't speak to dads from *their* point of view. They didn't go into detail about what it is like to be standing alongside the delivery table. They definitely didn't talk about what a birth partner can do to take an *active* role in labor, birth, and, especially, breastfeeding. Dads were expected to show up at the hospital and kind of figure it out from there.

To me, this just wasn't good enough. I felt like fathers needed more information and more pointers. I wanted birth partners to walk into the hospital feeling like a confident coach, like a true badass ready to take the labor and delivery unit by storm. I decided that I wanted to do more to prepare expectant fathers and birth partners everywhere for the experience of childbirth. That is how the Rocking Dads workshop series was born. I began meeting with soon-to-be dads in a classroom setting in order to educate and inspire them ahead of their parenting journey.

My passion for birth partnership began long before I became a father. When I was only nineteen years old, I attended my first birth. *Yes, you read that right: nineteen years old.* I was a surfer kid in Southern California at the time, completely unaware of the path my life was about to take. A dear family friend of mine had unexpectedly become pregnant. With the support of her family, she made the decision to carry the baby full-term and then put the baby up for adoption. This friend requested that I act as her coach and partner throughout the pregnancy and birth. Her father, Bruce, who was fighting esophageal cancer at the time, gave me his blessing to stand by his daughter. Bruce was an inspiration to me, a true role model in my life. My own dad had not been very present in my childhood, so I naturally looked to other men for guidance and support. The care and love I saw Bruce demonstrate with his wife and family of three daughters, even when he fell ill, was nothing short of amazing. He was there for his family, and I wanted to be there for his daughter. I felt honored and humbled that he wanted me to support her through the birth, and I took the job very seriously.

I attended Lamaze classes and a hospital tour with my expectant friend. We watched movies, went on walks, and laughed a ton. By the end of those ten months, she and I had taken our friendship to a new level, and I had learned a great deal. The birth was intense and incredible, especially for a nineteen-year-old surfer-musician! Can you imagine? It was in that moment that I fell in love with the act of birth assistance and birth partnership. The seed was planted. I saw how impactful it could be to have a supportive and well-informed birth partner by a mother's side. When I became a father to two daughters decades later, my belief in fostering strong birth partners was cemented.

I'm happy to report that I am still in touch with the family friend who gave birth all of those years ago. I am also in touch with the young lady who was born that day. Raised by adoptive parents, she has grown into an amazing adult woman. I love knowing that the beginning of her life led me to change gears in my own young life and move toward a career of supporting expectant parents.

My first early career move was to pursue a degree in radiological technology and eventually open up two ultrasound clinics. Later, after both of my daughters were born by emergency cesarean section, I decided to become a certified doula and a birth educator. These days, I partner with hundreds of couples every year, from the beginning of their pregnancy (at my ultrasound clinics) to the delivery of their baby (as a doula). Then I continue to support them after the birth as a lactation counselor and chief encourager. Can I tell you something? I love every minute of my job. And, I have learned a massive amount of information about pregnancy and giving birth over the years. My goal is to pass all of that learning on to you so that you feel confident and at ease when you walk into the hospital to welcome your baby into the world.

Let me give you a visual of how I see your role as an expectant father: Imagine yourself as a football quarterback during preseason. You're running drills and studying new plays. You and your team are devising a playbook. You're in it for the win, right? And you have a long and exciting season ahead of you. Bringing a baby into the world is no different. You have ten months of preparation, and then it is go time—for the next eighteen years. (Well, let's be real here, sometimes thirty-five years!) There's one thing I know for sure: you need a good coach to guide you. That is what I am here for. I'm ready to prepare you for parenting success.

About This Book

Let me fill you in on how I structured this guide. There are nine chapters, each with a different pregnancy-, childbirth-, or baby-related topic. Feel free to use this guide as a reference source. Skip around as you need, or read it cover to cover. If you read the whole thing, you will feel like you have attended one of my Rocking Dads courses. In the following nine chapters I present everything I share in my course. Here's a brief summary.

Chapter 1: The Basics. You've found out that you and your partner are expecting a baby. Congrats! Now I have a lot to teach you. In this chapter, I'll share all of the time lines, lingo, and pregnancy terms you need to know to be a well-informed pregnancy partner.

Chapter 2: Preparing Your Relationship and Yourself for Parenthood. You have ten months to get this parenting thing off to a good start. I'll give you tips on how to make your partnership with Mom stronger than ever and win the Partner of the Year Award. I'll also throw in some tips on how to prepare *yourself* for parenthood, which is going be a big transition for both of you.

Chapter 3: Planning and Packing for the Birth. You know how you make a list when you go to the grocery store or an itinerary when you go on vacation? Same thing here. I'm going to give you all the tools you need to plan out the birth the way that you and Mom want it to go. I'll also give you a list of things to purchase and pack for the hospital so that you feel fully equipped for the birth.

Chapter 4: Navigating Early Labor at Home. In this chapter, I talk about how to differentiate between prelabor, early labor, and active labor. Since most of early labor typically happens at home, I'll give you ideas on how to respond to Mom's needs and enjoy this special time together.

Chapter 5: Supporting Your Partner Through Active Labor. How do you know when it is time to go to the hospital, and what should you expect when you get there? I will give you the full rundown in this chapter and provide plenty of hints on how to support Mom during this intense yet beautiful experience.

Chapter 6: Pushing, Childbirth, and Beyond. Okay, guys, this is why you're here, right? To hear all about the actual birth. I will give you a GoPro-style description of what to expect in the delivery room and make you feel prepared to meet that sweet baby. I will also fill you in on what happens directly after the birth. We'll cover a lot in this chapter.

Chapter 7: Navigating C-Sections and Other Unusual Birth Circumstances. Although some cesarean sections are scheduled, many are not. I will give you tips on how to have a beautiful and memorable C-section experience, regardless of whether you are planning for one or not. I'll also give you advice on how to support your partner and yourself when dealing with any other birth complications or unforeseen scenarios.

Chapter 8: Your New Baby and Breastfeeding Basics. After that baby has emerged, and there has been plenty of skin-to-skin contact, the next focus will be breastfeeding. You can read up on nursing in this chapter so you can be your partner's number-one supporter as she and the baby figure out this new skill.

Chapter 9: Bringing Baby Home. Eventually, the hospital or birth center sends you and Mom home to do your thing. I'll give you suggestions on how to make this transition go smoothly, so that you and Mom don't feel like you are being thrown to the wolves.

A Few Other Notes About This Book

Throughout this book, you're often going to hear me refer to the birth parent as "Mom" and the birth partner as "Dad." I use these terms for the sake of simplicity. That being said, please know that the concepts and suggestions are applicable to *any* birth partnership: LGBTQ+ couples, adoptive parents, surrogate parents, birth partners who are friends or family members—all of the information in this book applies to you too. Take or leave the labels and soak up all of the suggestions that apply to your unique situation. Don't hesitate to reach out to me through social media or my website if you have questions that pertain to your specific circumstances.

I asked my friend and colleague Kirsten Brunner to be my coauthor, utilizing her twenty years of experience as a licensed professional counselor. She offers psychology-related pointers and suggestions throughout the book. Kirsten provides sanity-saving and relationship-strengthening hacks on her website, Baby Proofed Parents. Watch for these tips in the "Counselor Corner" sections in this book, accompanied by an image of Kirsten sitting in her counseling chair. Since Kirsten is also a mother of two young boys, she occasionally shares a "Mom Moment," in which she gives her personal perspective or experience.

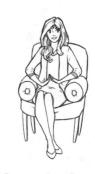

Counselor Corner

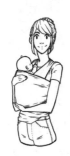

Mom Moment

You'll also see "Birth Guy Pointers" in every chapter because, believe me, I have plenty of insider tips to give. Look for the image of me in the classroom. Each time you see me by my whiteboard, I will be doling out hints and suggestions on how to win at the game of birth partnering. Additionally, there is a host of materials available for download at this book's website: http://www.newharbinger.com/41597. (See the very back of the book for details.)

By the time you finish this book, you will have all of the tools and information you need to be a fully prepared and fully confident birth partner. You'll be telling your partner, "I've got this. We've got this. We can do this, honey." Enjoy reading. Enjoy dreaming and planning for the birth of your baby. You are about to embark on the most amazing experience you've ever had. Kirsten and I will make sure you're prepared!

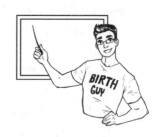

Birth Guy Pointers

CHAPTER 1

The Basics

What was it like when you first saw that positive pregnancy test? Exciting? Scary? Did you think, *Oh, crap! What did we do?* Regardless of whether your reaction was positive, negative, or a big, messy mixture, you're not alone. The expectant dads whom I work with experience a wide range of emotions, and all of them are completely normal. Bringing a baby into your life is a huge deal. Whether you and your partner have been trying to get pregnant for years, or this baby-to-be is a total surprise, the moment you're told you are going to be a parent is intense—and amazing. If you feel like you are on the brink of an incredible adventure, that is *because you are.*

In some ways, the journey to parenthood is like traveling to another country. There is an entire new language, full of pregnancy and parenting lingo, that you are suddenly expected to understand. You and your partner have to purchase and pack a collection of new gear and supplies. There are even customs and rituals to figure out as you go. And, like any good overseas adventure, you're not really sure how the trip is going to go until you get there.

But listen, don't worry. In this book, Kirsten and I are going to fill you in on everything you need to know for your journey. Similar to travel guides, we'll give you the lowdown on how to arrive at the port of parenthood in one piece. By the time you finish reading the last chapter you will be a Birth Guy–certified pregnancy, birth, and breastfeeding aficionado. Mom-to-be is going to be beyond impressed. Sound good? We've got you covered.

My first goal is to teach you all of the pregnancy basics, such as the common side effects of pregnancy, how to choose a doctor, physical limitations for Mom, and so on. I'm going to share with you all of the medical terms and lingo you need to know so that you can talk the talk and walk it, too.

Birth Guy Pointer: Pregnancy Apps. I encourage all of my dads to download a pregnancy app, such as BabyCenter, What to Expect, or The Bump. If you don't do smartphone apps, no biggie. You can go to one of the developer's websites and sign up for weekly emails. Just plug in your baby's due date and you'll begin receiving weekly messages in your inbox explaining:

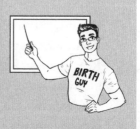

- the size of your baby in Mom's womb

- what is going on developmentally with the baby's body

- what physical sensations, discomforts, and changes Mom is most likely to be experiencing

- loads of other helpful information

After you have downloaded an app, or signed up for emails, make it a point to tune in and read the weekly updates. Your partner is going to love it when you say things like "Did you know that our baby is as big as an avocado right now?" or "I'm so sorry you feel tired and crappy. They say that you should start feeling better around week twelve or so. What can I do to help and support you right now?"

Okay, guys, let's sort through the nuts and bolts of the pregnancy adventure! When I meet with an expectant Mom and Dad for the first time, they usually greet me with a long list of questions. I answer what I can, and then I suggest that their doctor or midwife answer those that are more medical in nature. Below you will find a broad overview of everything you need to know for the next forty or so weeks. I've split the FAQs into four categories:

In the beginning: There is a lot to digest when you first launch into the conception and pregnancy experience. In this section, I'll address the most important things to know as you begin your journey toward parenthood.

All about Mom: A woman's body goes through an incredible transformation when she is carrying a baby. Here, I will fill you in on the anatomical changes, common side effects, and physical limitations that you and Mom should be aware of.

Bring in the experts: There are a lot of people who went through *a ton* of schooling and training to support you and your partner through pregnancy and birth. I'll share when it is appropriate to meet with each of them and how to pick the best practitioners for you.

Let's get this party started: During the second half of the pregnancy, the fun stuff really begins—baby showers, gender reveals, childbirth classes, and the nursery setup. Your full calendar and growing to-do list might feel overwhelming. I'll give you the lowdown so you can show up to the various activities with a smile on your face.

As you move through each of these sections, you might have specific questions that apply to your unique situation. Do not hesitate to contact your health care provider. We *all* want you to feel confident and informed on this amazing journey. Okay, here we go...

In the Beginning

You've just learned that you and your partner are going to be parents. Or maybe you're a few steps behind that and are trying to conceive. Regardless, I have answers to the questions that most of my dads and birth partners have when they meet with me early in the game.

Why do people say "expectant" parent instead of "expecting"? "Expectant" is just an adjective that means "eagerness" or "anticipation." Birth professionals tend to use this word when describing a person who is expecting a baby. But you know what? It means exactly the same thing as "expecting," so use whichever word you want! You're having a baby, and that's what matters.

How is a pregnancy confirmed? And when does it officially start? Most couples start with a standard home-pregnancy test: Mom-to-be pees on a stick, and within a few minutes, a little symbol pops up, indicating whether you are on your way to parenthood or not. Let me tell you, those little pee sticks have been a source of intense emotions for decades. These tests detect the amount of human chorionic gonadotropin (hCG), a strong indicator of pregnancy, that is present in urine. Mom's body starts pumping out this hormone immediately after the tiny egg attaches to the uterine wall, usually six days after fertilization has occurred. I always encourage couples to schedule an appointment with an ob-gyn or a midwife after they get that positive test. Your doctor might run an additional urine panel or blood panel to confirm the pregnancy. Your provider will probably schedule a transvaginal ultrasound around seven to eight weeks. This will allow you to get a first peek at your soon-to-be bundle.

Does pregnancy last nine or ten months? I'm confused. You're not alone… It is confusing. Pregnancy (or gestation) lasts approximately forty weeks, beginning on the first day of Mom's last period and ending on the day that the baby is born. Most babies arrive somewhere between thirty-seven and forty-two weeks, which equals nine or ten months, depending on how you measure months. To be honest, I like to throw out the month measurement and track a pregnancy using weeks.

The truth is that every pregnancy is different. A due date is really just an educated guess. Your baby might come early. She or he might come late. The experience is similar to when you're trying to get to happy hour during rush hour. You're not sure exactly when you'll get there, but as long as you eventually arrive, all is good. Am I right? It's the same with due dates. That baby will arrive when he or she arrives—don't get too caught up on the exact date.

How do you know if you are going to have twins? Or multiples? Are you allowed to freak out about this? The majority of the time, couples find out that they have two buns in the oven with the first transvaginal ultrasound, at seven or eight weeks. You'll see two little embryos and two flickering heartbeats instead of just one. Some couples see more than two. If this happens, can you freak out? Totally! It is normal to feel overwhelmed, scared out of your gourd, and thrilled—all at the same time. However, let me pause and share with you that this is a key moment for you as Mom's partner. Remaining calm and confident is the most important thing you can do for Mom. You want her to know that you're on her team and that you guys will do this thing together. Whether it is one, two, or five babies, you've got this. There are amazing resources out there for parents of multiples. You will have loads of support.

When are you out of the woods in regard to early miscarriage? Approximately 80 to 90 percent of all miscarriages (which are defined as a pregnancy loss in the first twenty weeks of gestation) occur in the first thirteen weeks of pregnancy (Wilcox et al. 1988). I encourage couples to not fixate on this time frame, however. We're looking for a paradigm shift here. Instead of focusing on risk or end dates, I like to tell Mom and Dad to focus on staying positive, healthy, and mentally strong. The best thing Mom can do during her pregnancy is take care of herself and her growing belly. Dad can help by encouraging Mom to focus on things she is in control of and then allowing her body to do the rest.

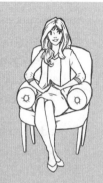

Counselor Corner: Anxiety During Pregnancy. Many moms notice an increase in their anxiety during pregnancy. Dads can also find themselves feeling worried about the health and safety of Mom and the baby. This makes sense—you are over-the-moon excited, and yet there are *so* many unknowns and uncertainties. If either of you is prone to anxiety or depression, it is common to see a spike in symptoms. I encourage clients to make more time than ever for calming, self-soothing activities: deep breathing, mindfulness, meditation, yoga, exercise, and positive affirmations. Focus on the things you can control and try to let go of the things you can't. Talk to loved ones. And please reach out to a counselor or your health care provider if your feelings of anxiety or depression feel over the top. The calmer both of you remain, the better it is for the pregnancy and your relationship.

Okay, I hear you about staying positive. Roger that. But what if our pregnancy does end in miscarriage? What do we do? About 20 percent of known pregnancies (that is, pregnancies confirmed with a test) end in miscarriage during the first trimester (Wilcox et al. 1988). Signs of miscarriage include menstrual-like cramps, abdominal pain, and bleeding. If Mom is experiencing any of these symptoms, she should definitely contact her health care provider as soon as possible. Most miscarriages are a onetime occurrence—the fact that Mom got pregnant in the first place is an excellent indicator that she will conceive again and go on to have a normal, healthy pregnancy. People often refer to babies born after a miscarriage as "rainbow babies." They are beautiful blessings that come after the storm. I have witnessed the delivery of many rainbow babies in my doula career, and they are some of the most joyful births. They are definitely little pots of gold.

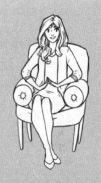

Counselor Corner: **Talking About Miscarriages.** Researchers say that the vast majority of early miscarriages are caused by chromosomal or chemical abnormalities in the baby, not anything that Mom or you did wrong. Even with this knowledge, a miscarriage can be really hard. It is a major loss, and there is grieving that goes along with that. Unfortunately, miscarriage tends to be a hush-hush topic—people don't talk about these losses nearly enough. I encourage clients to allow themselves time to grieve and process any emotions of sadness, disappointment, or anger that might arise. Talk to friends, talk to a counselor, and, most importantly, talk to each other. Supporting each other through these very normal emotions will help you to heal and move forward, when you are ready.

So when can we share the exciting news of our pregnancy with our family and friends? How about posting on social media? Every couple handles this differently. Some expectant parents can't bear to hold in the news—they share about the pregnancy as soon as they get the positive test. Other couples wait until the twenty-week mark. By this point, Mom is starting to show and she has had the midpregnancy ultrasound. I usually encourage clients to wait until after the first trimester, about twelve to sixteen weeks, to share their happy status with their crew. The same goes for social media. Even though you are bursting with excitement, it might be a good idea to hold off on the cute Instagram announcement until the pregnancy has progressed a bit.

All About Mom

I work with hundreds of expectant couples each year, and you know what never ceases to amaze me? The incredible transformation that a woman's body goes through in order to safely deliver a baby into this world. Nature is an awe-inspiring thing, isn't it? Keep reading to learn about the different internal renovations and possible side effects that Mom can expect to experience.

What is morning sickness? When does it start and end? Do all moms get it? How do you know if Mom has hyperemesis gravidarum? "Morning sickness" is a misnomer because it doesn't always happen in the morning. I like to refer to it as "anytime sickness." Some moms experience it throughout the day. Some moms never experience it. A small percentage of my clients suffer long into the third trimester. The majority of moms experience it between the six- and twelve-week points.

There are a lot of things that Mom can try if she is struggling with nausea: ginger pills and lollipops, B_6 vitamins, nausea wristbands, homeopathic remedies, and extra sleep. If the morning sickness becomes extreme and leads to excessive weight loss or dehydration, it is important to touch base with your health care provider. Mom might be diagnosed with hyperemesis gravidarum (extreme morning sickness), which could lead to hospitalization or IV hydration, or both. If Mom needs an IV, don't fret. It will make her feel so much better. A small percentage of moms are sent home with an anti-nausea-medication pump, similar to an insulin pump, so they can receive a continual flow of anti-nausea meds. The important thing is to get Mom stable so she can march on with the pregnancy and gain the appropriate amount of weight. Whether she has mild morning queasiness or hyperemesis gravidarum, Mom is going to need you to be her right-hand man and step in with a cold washcloth or a glass of water when needed.

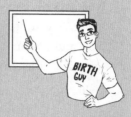
What about other pregnancy symptoms and side effects? Do dads experience any of these? Okay, you're probably going to get tired of me saying this, but every pregnancy is different. Some moms feel exhausted and emotional. Others feel like they've won the lottery and like they're ready to run a marathon. Most feel a mixture of highs and lows. And, the second pregnancy might be completely different from the first! Heartburn, strong emotions, food cravings, food aversions, sleep disturbances, and aches and pains are common side effects. There is a ton happening in Mom's body, and it makes sense that she is not always going to feel completely comfortable.

Do dads and birth partners experience some of these side effects? Sure! I see dads experience emotional ups and downs, food cravings, and other vicarious symptoms. This is a big adventure for you as well, and it is natural that you are going to be all over the place as you prepare for parenthood. The important thing is that you and Mom stay connected, share about how you are feeling, practice patience with each other, and offer support whenever you can.

Mom Moment: Mom's Changing Body. Weight gain and body changes are obvious side effects of pregnancy. If Mom is healthy and at an average weight before pregnancy, she will typically gain twenty-five to thirty-five pounds in order to support the growing baby. While some moms enjoy their new curves, others feel self-conscious about their expanding middle and worry about whether they will be able to lose the weight after the pregnancy. The most powerful thing you can do in these moments is to reassure Mom that she is beautiful and that her body is doing exactly what it is supposed to be doing: expanding to meet the needs of the 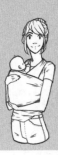 baby. Occasionally, dads will share with me that they do not find their wife's pregnancy attractive or sexy. Some partners admit that they find breastfeeding a turnoff. I politely encourage them to keep their distaste to themselves and to try to tune in to the beauty of what their partner's body is accomplishing. Mom needs support and acceptance as her body works hard to support a new life.

Tell me about this ongoing remodel in Mom's abdomen. What is the placenta, umbilical cord, and amniotic sac, among other things? "Remodeling" is a good way to describe what is happening inside Mom's body. There will be tons of expanding and building as the baby begins to grow. The easiest way for me to explain what is going on is with an illustration.

An Inside Look at Mom:
Before & During Pregnancy

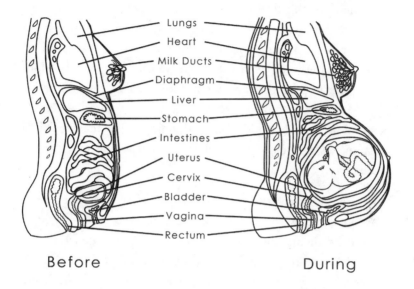

Lungs
Heart
Milk Ducts
Diaphragm
Liver
Stomach
Intestines
Uterus
Cervix
Bladder
Vagina
Rectum

Before   During

There are some key things to pay attention to with the illustration above. Notice how Mom's stomach and intestines get squeezed against the top of her abdomen. No wonder she experiences some heartburn and constipation! The same is true with her bladder: the baby rests right on top of it, so don't be surprised if Mom needs to head to the restroom more frequently. And check out what's happening to her spine. It supports a whole heck of a lot of weight in front. This causes Mom to walk a little differently, possibly with a slight waddle.

You may also notice a few additions to Mom's abdomen. Of course, there is a baby in there, but there's also an amniotic sac surrounding the baby and protecting it with fluid. That ropelike thing is the umbilical cord, which nourishes your little one. I will cover all of these aspects of pregnancy in more detail later in the book.

When will Mom be able to feel the baby move? When will I be able to see or feel the baby move? Mom should be able to feel the baby move sometime between sixteen and twenty-five weeks. Most moms describe this feeling as being a little like gas bubbles at first. It's an exciting moment in the pregnancy, especially if this is your first baby. Most dads and partners don't get to feel, or see, the baby move until after week twenty. If you're waiting for a little handprint or footprint to peek through Mom's skin, you'll be waiting a long time. Mom's body provides several layers of cushion between the baby and the outside world. This cushioning causes the baby's kicks and punches to look kind of like an alien poking out from her insides. Pretty cool, huh?

How about activity and exercise? Yoga? Most doctors and midwives not only say that activity and exercise are okay, they highly recommend them. The same goes for yoga. The more Mom takes care of her body, the better it is for the pregnancy and birth. Exercise promotes strength and endurance, both of which will be helpful during the birth and postpartum period. Prenatal yoga is amazing for relaxation, strength building, and positive visualization, which are also helpful during the birth. I have two cautionary statements, however:

1. Mom should always get doctor or midwife approval before embarking on a strenuous exercise program.

2. If Mom is not feeling well, she might not be up for exercising. Don't pressure or shame her if she doesn't feel like being super active. Even gentle walks around the block are great for Mom and are an excellent way for you and her to connect and bond during pregnancy.

How about sex during pregnancy? Absolutely, yes! You should double-check this one with your doctor or midwife first, but in most cases, sexual activity is encouraged. Let's list off the reasons why:

- Sex releases pleasurable hormones such as oxytocin and endorphins that can help Mom feel more relaxed and help her to sleep better.

- Intimacy is a great way to connect and strengthen your bond before the baby arrives.

- Sex and intimacy provide opportunities to practice perineal massage and prepare Mom for delivery. (We'll discuss this more in chapter 4.)

- Sex is fun, right? Need I say more?

Counselor Corner: Sex and Touch During Pregnancy.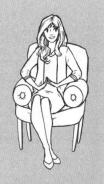
Intimacy is a topic that comes up frequently in my pre-natal and postpartum counseling sessions with couples. Some women feel more beautiful and sexual than ever during the pregnancy, and even after the birth. Other moms notice a decrease in their libido due to hormonal fluctuations or a lack of energy. It is important to follow Mom's lead and not pressure her into making love if she is not feeling in the mood. I encourage couples to find other ways to be intimate and feel close: cuddling, massage, or sitting close on the sofa. Brian urges couples to practice slow dancing, which is also a great activity to do during labor. Turn on some smooth music and tune in to each other. Switch your objective from sexual activity to connecting with Mom and helping her to relax. This will benefit the pregnancy and increase intimacy.

Are there things Mom should avoid eating? Any other dangers?
Sorry if I'm sounding like a broken record, but I encourage you to

touch base with Mom's doctor or midwife on this topic. The recommendations for foods and drinks to avoid are always changing. Here is the standard list of no-nos that I often hear from doctors:

- unpasteurized dairy (including most stinky cheeses, such as blue cheese and brie)

- deli meats and processed meats, because they might contain a harmful bacteria called listeria

- salad bar items, which might contain bacteria if they haven't been appropriately washed or kept cool

- raw fish or undercooked meat (Yup, sushi is out the window, folks.)

- more than two hundred milligrams of caffeine (approximately one to two cups of coffee) a day

- high-mercury fish such as shark, swordfish, or albacore tuna

- alcohol (beer, wine, cocktails...you name it)

Okay, did I just list off all of Mom's favorites? I know. That stinks. However, I notice that most moms are more than happy to give up these items temporarily for the sake of the pregnancy and the baby's health. You know how you can support Mom? Join her in abstaining from some, or all, of these items. She'll love that you are making a few sacrifices along with her, and both of you will arrive at the finish line of birth healthy and in great shape.

There are other things that Mom's provider will probably encourage her to avoid, such as changing and cleaning kitty-litter boxes, going on roller coasters, and taking most medications (unless specifically approved). Ask the doc for the list of no-nos at the first appointment. It won't be a long list, but it will be an important one to pay attention to.

Bring in the Experts

Doctors, midwives, and doulas, oh my! When you become pregnant, you have a lot of options for who, when, where, and what you choose for pregnancy support and birth services. Here's the lowdown on how to seek support from the many professionals who want to assist you.

When does Mom need to see the doctor for the first time? How often should she go? Should Dad go to every appointment? If Mom has an ob-gyn or midwife with whom she is established and feels comfortable, she'll want to call that person and schedule an appointment as soon as she gets the positive home-pregnancy test. Office staff will often ask for the start date of Mom's last period so they can approximate the baby's due date and schedule Mom's first appointment according to that time frame.

As for dads and birth partners attending appointments—*hell, yes*, you should attend! Go to as many appointments as you can. Prenatal appointments are a great way to learn about the pregnancy, bond with your partner, get to know the doctor, and hear your little baby's heartbeat. Putting aside time to show up at these appointments will let Mom know that you care, which in turn will help her feel like both of you are on the same page.

How do you decide whether to use a doctor or a midwife? How about whether a hospital, birth center, or home birth is right for you? There are so many choices, right? But they are great choices. I'm glad that so many of my clients get to choose the birthing environment that is best for them. If you are hoping to use medical insurance for prenatal care and baby delivery, I recommend that you contact your insurance company and find out exactly what is covered. This will help you to narrow your options. Next, think about both of your personalities and preferences, and then have a discussion about the best birthing environment for Mom. The good news is that I have been seeing a trend of birthing locations utilizing each other's best practices and blending them. Some hospitals have introduced birth centers in which midwives and doctors work alongside each other. More and more independent birth centers are popping up, and some have the medical technology and facilities of a hospital. I advise you to see what is available in your community and to take a few tours. Here's some information to help you explore your options based on your personalities:

- Do you and your partner love freedom and space? Do you avoid traditional Western medicine in favor of natural or homeopathic treatments? Do you want as much one-on-one time with each other as possible during the birth? Do you love being in your home more than any other place? Is seeking adventure kind of your thing?

  If so, you might want to work with a midwife *and deliver your baby* at home.

Birth Guy Pointer: Finding the Right Provider. Let me tell you something that is *even more important* than scheduling with an ob-gyn or midwife after the positive pregnancy test: finding an ob-gyn or midwife whom you like and trust. Believe me, I hang out in delivery rooms with plenty of doctors and new parents, and I can tell whether there is a 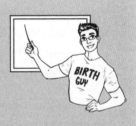 love connection or not between the different parties. Things go a heck of a lot more smoothly if everyone is on the same page. Finding the right provider is sort of like dating: you might need to see who's out there before you settle on one. Feel free to shop around for ob-gyns or midwives until you find a match. Look at their websites, and go to their "meet the doc" sessions ready with questions. Even if you've already seen a provider for a first session, you can always switch to someone else. It is so important that you feel a rapport with the person who is going to deliver your baby—it will make the experience *that* much more successful.

- Do you and your partner like the continual flow of information that medical technology and testing can provide? Even if you're planning for a natural birth, do you like the thought of doctors and interventions being close by? Is Mom planning on taking advantage of pain-reduction options, such as an epidural? Has there been a high-risk pregnancy or medical trauma in the past? Do you like the idea of being taken care of for a few days before heading home?

  If so, you might want to work with a doctor *and deliver your baby* at a hospital.

- Are your personalities a combination of the above? Do you like the idea of going for a natural birth but want basic monitoring close at hand? Do you want the homeyness of a home birth, but you don't want to deliver the baby in your own home? Do you dislike hospitals? Would you prefer to bring the baby home as soon as possible?

  If so, you might want to work with a midwife *or a* doctor *and deliver your baby* at a birth center.

What exactly does a doula do? When is it helpful or appropriate to work with a doula? Doula is a Greek word that means "woman's servant." Centuries of doulas supporting women in childbirth have proven that a helper can have a positive impact on the labor process. In fact, research has shown that doula-assisted mothers are four times less likely to have a low-birth-weight baby, two times less likely to experience a birth complication involving themselves or their baby, and significantly more likely to successfully initiate breastfeeding (Gruber, Cupito, and Dobson 2013). Those are pretty great outcomes, right?

These days, a doula not only supports Mom during the birth, but also acts as a liaison between the parents and the medical personnel. Doulas advocate for Mom and Dad and help them to make their birth plan a reality. I take things a step further in my work as a doula (or "dude'la," as some people like to call me). I meet with the couple several times before the birth and do relationship-building exercises with Mom and Dad. I lead them on a hospital tour and encourage them to take my childbirth classes and any others courses that the hospital might offer. When Mom goes into labor, I am there by the couple's side. I might be there for six hours or for thirty-six hours, but I don't leave until the baby is latching on to Mom's breast.

Yes, I am a man, and I have sort of broken the mold of the typical doula, but I see my gender as a plus that helps me to connect with Dad and involve him even more in the birth. If you are considering hiring a doula, here are the questions you might want to ask yourself:

- Is this your first birth?

- Has Mom experienced birth traumas or other medical or hospital traumas in the past?

- Are either of you feeling especially anxious about the birth?

- Do either of you have difficulty communicating your wants and needs with your doctor?

- Do you want support and coaching so you can be the best birth partner you can be?

If you answered yes to any of the above questions, then you might want to consider hiring a doula. It is an investment that will be well worth it when you get to labor day and it's time to meet your baby.

What are genetic tests, and should we do them? Will there be other tests or screens? Things have changed a lot since my first daughter was born more than a decade ago. It seems like doctors can test for everything now. Whether or not you do these tests is up to you and Mom. I encourage couples to talk to their doctor or midwife about which tests are available, which ones are recommended, which ones are standard, and which ones are optional and possibly more invasive. Your health care provider might recommend that you consult with a genetic counselor if there are medical or genetic concerns in either of your families. After you have gathered info about these tests, go home, talk with your partner, and choose the path that feels right for both of you.

When do we choose a pediatrician—that is, a doctor for kids?
Most couples start thinking about choosing a pediatrician sometime during the second trimester. You might be thinking, Why the heck do we need a pediatrician? We don't even have a kid yet! Right. I hear you. However, most new parents are encouraged to take their baby for a checkup within the first week or so after the birth, regardless of where the birth occurred. You can ask neighbors and friends with kids for recommendations. You can also check online reviews to find someone whose views jive with yours. You and your family will potentially have a relationship with this doc for the next thirteen to eighteen years, so here are some tips for choosing the right one:

- What is the doctor's availability? Is it hard to get an appointment? Does the doctor have weekend or on-call hours, or both? What happens if there is a medical emergency?

- Does the doctor accept your insurance? (This is important!) If not, what are typical fees?

- What is the office like? Is it clean and up-to-date? Is the front-desk staff polite and friendly?

- Do you like the doctor's personality? Does she or he seem culturally sensitive to the needs of your family? Does he or she have kids?

- How long has the doctor been in practice?

- Do the policies and practices of the office fit with your views? What is the doctor's policy on immunizations? Is the doctor's practice breastfeeding friendly?

A great way to answer these questions is to go to a "meet the doc" night, which many pediatricians offer. The practice's website should offer the date, time, and location of these meet and greets. And, of course, you should visit the actual office. You can get a good feel for the practice by sitting in its office space for a while and visiting with the doctor.

What is an ultrasound? When do you have the first ultrasound? Do ultrasounds harm the baby? Ultrasounds, also called sonograms, are used to determine the gender of your baby and to check for any abnormalities in the baby's development. Ultrasound imaging uses sound waves to produce pictures of the inside of the body. It is widely considered to be a safe and noninvasive procedure. The person carrying out the scans (a sonographer) will follow all the appropriate guidelines to ensure that you and your baby are safe. Another plus is that ultrasounds don't use ionizing radiation, as x-ray imaging does. This makes them well suited for taking good, long looks at your growing baby.

Typically, a doctor will do a transvaginal ultrasound around six to eight weeks to confirm the pregnancy and to take a first look at your tiny baby. During this procedure, the doctor inserts an ultrasound probe into Mom's vagina because the baby is too tiny to view through the abdominal lining. This first ultrasound is when you will see the heartbeat flickering! It is really exciting. The next medical scan will be between eighteen and twenty-two weeks. If you haven't learned the sex of your baby before now, this will be your opportunity. During this scan, the sonographer will also measure the baby's organs and features, looking for any abnormalities. At BabyVision Ultrasound, my ultrasound center in San Antonio, we determine gender at fifteen weeks. This may be an option for you too. If you want to see your baby in 3D/4D/HD Live, it is best to go to the ultrasound clinic at twenty-eight weeks, when the baby is a little chubbier. If Mom weighs more than 225 pounds, I suggest waiting until thirty-two weeks so that the baby is bigger and more visible.

How big is the baby at each step of the way? The best way to illustrate this is using fruit. Yup, fruit. Here is a chart to show you how big your little bundle is at different intervals during Mom's pregnancy.

How big is baby?

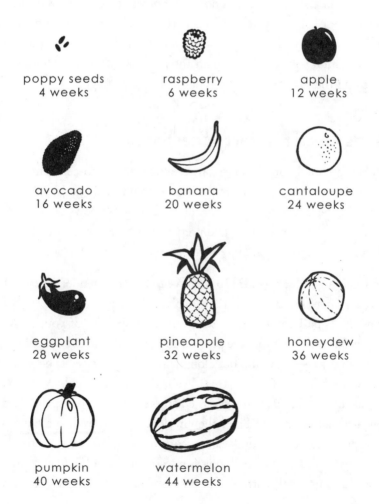

poppy seeds
4 weeks

raspberry
6 weeks

apple
12 weeks

avocado
16 weeks

banana
20 weeks

cantaloupe
24 weeks

eggplant
28 weeks

pineapple
32 weeks

honeydew
36 weeks

pumpkin
40 weeks

watermelon
44 weeks

When do we find out the sex or gender of the baby? Should we wait until the birth? For couples who want to know the sex of their baby, they find out during the midpregnancy ultrasound, usually performed between sixteen and twenty weeks, unless the baby is feeling shy and won't let the ultrasound technician get a good look at the genitals. Some couples find out the sex of their baby through noninvasive prenatal testing as early as ten weeks. This blood test, which looks for pieces of the male sex chromosome in the expectant mother's blood, can also detect Down syndrome and a few other chromosomal conditions. Some couples wait until the birth to find out the sex. There is no wrong or right way to find out the sex of your baby. If you and your partner are more traditional and like surprises, you might want to wait until the birth for the big reveal. But if you two like to plan and know what is on the horizon, learning the sex early on might be the best way to go.

Let's Get This Party Started

When a baby is on the horizon, everyone wants to celebrate and help you get ready. There are parties to attend, there is shopping to do, and there is a nursery to decorate. The good news is that you can shape these gatherings and preparations in a way that feels like a fit for you and Mom. Here is the scoop on what is ahead.

What is a gender reveal? Do we have to do it? A gender reveal is a twenty-first-century trend that involves throwing a big party—or having a small gathering—to announce the gender of your baby-to-be. Most of the time, the parents-to-be are also in the dark about the baby's sex—they find out along with everyone else at the party. How the heck do they do this? Well, the couple usually asks the ultrasound technician to write the baby's sex on a slip of paper and put it in an envelope. Then the envelope is delivered to a bakery that prepares a blue or pink cake accordingly, or to a friend who fills a box with pink or blue balloons to release, or to a golf ball company that fills a golf ball with blue or pink powder. The couple cuts into the cake, or releases the balloons, or hits the golf ball, the color is revealed, and everyone cheers. If this sounds like fun to you, I say make the party happen. This is the only time in your life when everyone will be cheering and crying about food coloring, and that is pretty priceless.

What are baby showers? Do dads have to go? Baby showers can be traced back to the 1950s when we entered the age of shopping. Women would gather to "shower" Mom-to-be with nursery items and baby gifts. These showers were about cuteness to the max: the decor, the cake, the games, and the gifts. These days, I've been seeing a trend toward couple's showers. Both Mom and Dad get to come. Things are a little less cute and a little more rowdy, but one thing is the same: you get showered with a lot of the stuff you need to care for your new little one. So…the more showers, the better. Am I right? Stock up on those diapers and onesies, guys. You're going to need them.

Should we register for baby stuff? Registering means that you and Mom walk into a store that sells baby gear (or log on to a website), choose the items that you like, and then add them to a master list that your friends and family can select gifts from. Most stores give you this really cool scanner gun that you can just zap the bar codes with. Sounds like fun, right? Whether you and your partner decide to register is up to you. Most couples like to do this so they can choose the colors for the nursery or the brand of bottles they like. Registering is also a great way to make sure you get everything on your list instead of fifty newborn outfits and nothing else. In chapter 9, I provide a list of things you might want to consider purchasing. Going to a baby store and registering is a great opportunity to have a date night with Mom. Better yet, plan a double date! Ask a couple who recently had a baby to join you. They can point out the things that you really need and tell you to skip the things that are just fluff.

Should we go to childbirth classes or other classes? What are the benefits? There are a ton of things that we learn by trial and error in life: how to cook, how to change a tire, how to romance a partner, how to pour a beer without a bunch of foam on top. You try things out, you fail, and you try again. Let me tell you something: Childbirth, infant care, and breastfeeding are not activities that you have to go into blindly. There are classes, awesome classes, that will teach you all of the basics and help you to feel prepared. In fact, that is what this book is all about: everything that I teach in my Rocking Dads class is sandwiched between these two covers. By the time you've read the last page, you will have completed my basic childbirth and breastfeeding course for birth partners. If your hospital or birth center provides free or low-cost classes, I encourage you to take advantage of them as well. If you've never cared for a baby before, infant-care and baby-soothing classes can be lifesavers. You will still be learning as you go, and occasionally you'll feel like you are failing, because all of us parents have felt that way, but you will feel more prepared if you do a few crash courses beforehand.

When should Mom stop working? How about Dad? This is another one of those questions with an answer specific to the individual. Everyone is a little different. Some moms like to work right up to the minute they go into labor. Their water breaks at the office and they're out the door! Others finish up work a few weeks early in order to get the nursery ready and get nice and chill before the birth. If there are any pregnancy complications, the doctor or midwife might require Mom to wrap up work several weeks before the birth. And then there are those rare occasions when the doctor will put Mom on bed rest for medical reasons, so going to work will be out of the question. Talk to your doctor, talk to Mom, consider how strenuous her job is and how much maternity leave she has, and make a decision that feels good to both of you. The same goes for Dad's work. Most of the dads and birth partners I work with like to save up their parental leave for after the baby arrives. That way, they can be at home to support Mom and spend as much time with their new little bundle.

I'm feeling overwhelmed by all this info! Help! Hey, listen, take a big breath. I don't expect you to soak in all of this information at once. Open the book up as needed. Remember, you'll figure out a lot of this stuff as you go. At the end of each chapter, I'm going to leave you with my "BG Final Shots," three pointers designed to give you the winning edge in the game of birth partnering. Even if you only read these, they will make you a champion.

BG FINAL SHOTS

✔ *Every Mom and every pregnancy is unique, kind of like a snowflake or a fingerprint.* Avoid comparing your experience to others—your journey is special and different. I know I sound like a Hallmark commercial, but it's true. That said, always check in with Mom's doctor or midwife if you have specific questions or concerns pertaining to the pregnancy.

✔ *This is a great time to start building your village.* You and Mom do not have to figure everything out on your own. Talk to other new parents, health care providers, trusted friends, birth educators, counselors, baby-store employees, and anyone else who will listen, support, and encourage you. You're probably surrounded by people who love to talk about babies and want to help. Tell them to hook you up!

✔ *You have forty weeks, give or take a few, to prepare Mom and yourself for childbirth and parenting.* That's plenty of time! Enjoy this special space as a couple and go at your own pace while making the many decisions ahead of you. *You're on your way, Dad!*

CHAPTER 2

Preparing Your Relationship and Yourself for Parenthood

Taylor and Samantha met in college. After four years of dating, they went window-shopping for engagement rings, but Taylor kept finding reasons to put off proposing. When friends questioned him about his hesitation, Taylor mentioned Sam's "neediness" and explained that he often felt smothered by her anxiety. Sam had her own concerns—Taylor didn't drink alcohol every day, but when he did drink, he usually went overboard. According to Sam, Taylor wasn't necessarily "the happiest drunk." Sam also complained that she was the only one who did any housework in the small apartment they shared.

All of these concerns melted away when they found out that Sam was pregnant. Although neither voiced it, they both believed that a baby could add that extra something that was lacking in their relationship. They excitedly attended the first doctor's appointment together and became even more giddy when they found out they were having a little girl.

Unfortunately, the distraction from their relationship woes was short-lived. Sam's anxiety about Taylor's drinking and the upcoming birth began to build. When she turned to Taylor for support, she felt like he was distant and cold. Taylor admitted that he was feeling nervous about becoming a dad. He felt like Sam was nagging him more than ever, and he confessed to sneaking in free time and brews with his buddies whenever he could. He wasn't sure what life would be like after the baby arrived. When Sam's water broke at thirty-nine weeks, the couple headed to the hospital feeling wary about what lay ahead of them.

Carlos and Jane had been married for seven years and had been trying to conceive a baby for four. After going through two rounds of in vitro fertilization, they were thrilled to learn they were going to be parents. In spite of her excitement, Jane was surprised to notice feelings of depression surfacing during the first trimester. She had struggled with depression in the past but didn't expect to feel blue during a pregnancy she so desperately wanted. Carlos encouraged Jane to see a counselor and eventually attended a few sessions with her.

During the couples sessions, multiple concerns came up. Carlos confessed that he was worried about their finances and Jane's desire to quit working after the baby arrived. Jane shared that she was feeling insecure about her changing body and wondered if Carlos was still attracted to her. Both expressed anxiety about the ways that their relationship would change after the baby arrived. The marital counselor worked with Jane to address the symptoms of depression and prepare her for the postpartum period. The counselor also helped them to process their relationship concerns and to make a plan for supporting each other before and after the baby arrived.

By the end of the third trimester, Jane and Carlos were feeling more in love and more connected than ever. When they headed to the hospital for a scheduled C-section, they felt strong in their relationship and ready for the adventures ahead.

I worked with both of these couples as a doula. When I met up with Jane and Carlos at the hospital for their C-section, they were pumped and ready to take on whatever came their way. Their relationship wasn't perfect, and both of them had concerns, but they felt like they had each other's backs and had a plan for moving forward. I continued to see this strength in their relationship during my postpartum visits with them. They were affectionate and patient with each other, even when they were tired or struggling.

Taylor and Sam were another story. Their birth went smoothly but there was noticeable tension in the delivery room. When I went for postpartum visits, the baby was doing okay, but Mom and Dad seemed distant and irritated with each other. I encouraged them to address the issues in their relationship before their ability to happily co-parent and cohabitate declined to the point of no return.

I tell you these stories to illustrate a topic that rarely gets mentioned in pregnancy manuals. In fact, this portion of childbirth prep, what I call relationship strength training, is often skipped altogether. And yet Kirsten and I agree that it is one of the most important skill sets to develop when gearing up to become a parent. You and your partner will have a thousand-times-better birth experience if you do the work to strengthen and maintain your relationship *before* you enter the delivery room. I guarantee it.

Why do we feel so strongly about this prep? There is a saying that I use a lot when talking to expectant couples: *you can't build a house on sand*. Clichéd as it sounds, it is spot on when you are starting a family. When you and your partner have a baby, you are introducing a brand-new dynamic to your relationship. You are expanding your dyad into a triad (or maybe even a larger grouping, if you're expecting twins or multiples). That is a big deal! If there are any weak spots in your relationship, you might find yourselves collapsing under the weight of parenthood. So instead, let's start with a sturdy and strong foundation. What does this mean? Take a look at your relationship with your partner (and I mean *a good look*) and determine if there are any areas that could use some work. Here are some questions that I usually ask my clients to think about:

- Are there any unresolved issues or grudges that need to be addressed and worked through?

- How do the two of you handle conflict? Do you scream and fight? Shut down completely? Hold resentments for days? Conflict is a normal and healthy part of being in a relationship, but how you handle it makes all the difference.

- How do you spend time together as a couple and make your relationship a priority?

- What state are your finances in? Is your home ready for the addition of a baby?

- Are there any addictions or unhealthy behaviors that need to be addressed?

- Are either of you prone to anxiety? How about depression? What do each of you do for self-care?

I could go on and on, but you get the idea. The nine to ten months of pregnancy are a great time to thoroughly examine your partnership and do some maintenance. I often recommend that couples see a therapist to work through any unresolved issues. Even if you decide against counseling, the exercises in this chapter will help you to address and strengthen any weak areas. Young children, especially newborns, feed off the energy in the home, so you want the energy to be as positive and healthy as possible. Again, you're not going for perfection or zero conflict. You're just going for a strong, sturdy foundation so that when you get tired or testy with each other, you can weather the storm.

Strengthening Trust and Intimacy Through the Trimesters

One way to fortify your relationship before the baby enters the picture is to respond to Mom's physical and emotional needs during the various phases of the pregnancy. As I emphasized in the last chapter, every woman experiences pregnancy in slightly different ways. It is important to take Mom's lead and respond to her unique symptoms and needs, as called for. However, there are some common pregnancy norms that *most* couples can count on. Over the next few pages, I give suggestions for how you can be Mom's biggest supporter every step of the way as she counts down to the baby's arrival. The result will be increased trust and intimacy during a really exciting time of your life.

Counselor Corner: Pre-baby Counseling. I see a steady stream of expectant couples in my counseling practice, many of whom are referred by Brian. Couples who are about to have a baby are some of my favorite clients to work with. I view this work as being similar to premarital counseling. You're embarking on a life-changing adventure, so why not do as much as you can to feel prepared and united as a couple.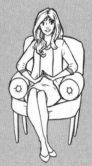

Research shows that relationship counseling can be extremely effective. A 2003 review found that couples who participated in premarital programs experienced a 30-percent increase in marital success over those who did not participate (Carroll and Doherty). These couples reported improved communication, better conflict-management skills, higher dedication to one's mate, greater emphasis on the positive aspects of a relationship, and improved overall relationship quality. Pretty good results, huh? In a 2010 study of 134 "chronically and seriously distressed" married couples, 48 percent showed clinically significant improvement when surveyed five years after having received marital therapy (Christensen et al.). My guess is that this percentage would be even higher if couples initiated counseling before they were seriously distressed.

In the pre-baby counseling I do with couples, we work on conflict management, focusing on recognizing each other's strengths and reserving plenty of patience and kindness for each other. Counseling sessions are a great opportunity to address any anxieties or mood irregularities that are coming up for Mom or Dad. Oftentimes, medical insurance will cover the cost of the sessions. Don't be afraid to suggest counseling to your partner if you think the two of you might benefit.

The First Trimester—Weeks One Through Twelve

What's going on physically: Hormones such as estrogen and progesterone are coursing through Mom's system as the pregnancy is established. She doesn't look pregnant yet, but she feels pregnant with all of her being. She might experience morning sickness, mood swings, and extreme fatigue.

What's going on emotionally: It is common for Mom to feel an increase in anxiety during the first trimester. Worries about miscarriage or other pregnancy complications can be persistent. Moms often ask, "Is this real? Am I really pregnant?" Mom might feel a loss of control—there are suddenly things that she can't eat, drink, or do, not to mention the fact that she can't really see what's happening inside of her. Captain Baby is suddenly driving the bus!

Concrete actions for Dad

- Listen to Mom and show empathy. ("I'm sorry you are feeling so drained. I imagine that it is exhausting to grow a baby. Why don't you go rest while I finish up the dishes.")

- Expect your partner to be more emotional and tired than usual. Give ample reassurance and encouragement. ("I hear you about feeling worried. We can't see what that little baby is doing in there, right? But you are doing an amazing job of taking care of yourself. Let's focus on trusting your body to take care of this baby. We'll be heading to the doctor for another checkup soon.")

- Help out with household chores and other duties whenever you can.

- Encourage Mom to focus on the things she *can* control: how she structures her day, how she pampers herself, how she allows for extra rest, and so on.

The Second Trimester—Weeks Thirteen Through Twenty-Seven

What's going on physically: Many expectant moms enjoy the second trimester the most. Energy often returns and the pregnancy starts to show. Physical symptoms such as nausea and heartburn are often more manageable. You get a good look at your baby during an ultrasound, and you and Mom can feel the baby moving in the womb. The excitement really starts to settle in.

What's going on emotionally: Although the second trimester can be enjoyable, it can still be a time of uncertainty and anxiety for Mom. Parents often face decisions about which medical and genetic tests to undergo. This can be confusing and daunting. Mom might feel insecure about her rapidly changing body and the pregnancy weight she is gaining.

Concrete actions for Dad

- Let the compliments about Mom's beauty flow. Her body is growing a baby! Let her know that you think she's gorgeous, inside and out.

- Talk through any difficult choices about testing or the pregnancy that the two of you have to make. Verbally processing any worries or decisions can often help to alleviate anxiety. Consult with your doctor or midwife when needed.

- Initiate brainstorming sessions about nursery decor and baby names.

- Get out and about when Mom is feeling good: Suggest date nights and small road trips if Mom is feeling up for it. Go to your favorite baby store and set up a registry.

- Don't be surprised if Mom still struggles with fatigue or other symptoms. Continue to be her right-hand mate.

The Third Trimester—Week Twenty-Eight Through to the Birth

What's going on physically: Mom and the baby are in the home-stretch now. Mom might begin experiencing more difficulty sleeping and face challenges with getting around. Heartburn, congestion, and insomnia are common complaints during this period. Baby showers, more frequent doctor visits, and shopping trips can keep both of you busy.

What's going on emotionally: At this point in the pregnancy, some moms hit a wall. They're thinking, *When is this baby going to get out of me already!*? Mom might also complain about "baby brain," a fogginess that makes her more forgetful and absentminded. Experts debate whether baby brain is really a thing, but most moms will argue that it is. My theory is that sleep disturbances and a developing maternal instinct interrupt usual brain functioning. Toward the end of the third trimester, most moms also start to nest, which can involve compulsive cleaning, endless organizing, impulsive shopping, or voracious purging in an effort to get ready for the baby.

Concrete Actions for Dad

- Continue to support Mom in whatever ways she finds helpful. Encourage naps if she is tired. Prop pillows behind her if she's bothered by heartburn. Help out around the house as much as possible.

- Help Mom keep her eye on the prize by reminding her that the birth is around the corner, and that she is doing great. ("You've amazed me the last eight months. Our baby is coming soon—we're almost there! Hang in there and tell me how I can help.")

- Exercise extra patience if Mom is experiencing any fogginess, forgetfulness, or other baby brain symptoms.

- In chapter 3, I give you a list of helpful things to bring to the hospital. If you haven't already, now is the time to shop. Gather what you need to be a fully prepared birth partner.

- In between shopping and nursery prep, make sure to spend plenty of quality time together as a couple. You will soon be transitioning from a couple to a family, so enjoy your days with just the two of you.

HEY, WHAT ABOUT DAD'S NEEDS?

You might be thinking, *What about me? I'm going through a massive life transition as well. Why is all of the focus on Mom?* You're absolutely right, Dad. You might not be experiencing the physiological or hormonal changes that Mom is going through, but you're still facing changes in your partner, your relationship, and your life. Sometimes dads report feelings of depression, anxiety, or moodiness. If Mom is really struggling with the pregnancy, it can be stressful and overwhelming for Dad. I encourage birth partners to take just as much time for self-care as Mom. This is a big deal for you, as well, Dad. Take care of you! Birth Guy orders.

Keeping the Love Alive in Your Changing Relationship

I started working with Mitzi and Korben soon after they discovered they were pregnant with twins. They wanted as much support as possible while preparing for the double-trouble that was brewing in Mitzi's belly. While working with them on labor techniques and breastfeeding skills, I noticed that they were completely focused on the content that I was teaching, but they were not very focused on each other. They sat on opposite sides of the room and weren't a bit affectionate. When I asked them about it, they laughed. "We've been together for over five years, Brian. The honeymoon period is over, right?" Mitzi insisted. "We love each other but we're not real lovey-dovey or anything."

"If I had my way, there would definitely be some more love-making happening. Wink, wink." Korben chimed in. "But, hey, I think it's normal for things to slow down after you've been together for a while. I'll tell you one thing, we're both feeling totally in love with these babies we're about to have."

My suspicions about Mitzi and Korben were confirmed. They were completely focused on the twins that they were about to have, not their relationship. All good, right? Well, sort of. Your relationship came before the baby, and hopefully it will be there for a long time after. If you make your union, and the romance in your union, a priority, you will be a stronger parenting team in the long run.

MAKE A LIST OF TEN

When couples get pregnant, often they have been together for a while. As Mitzi and Korben confirmed, they've usually passed the honeymoon stage and entered a more comfortable, sometimes even boring, stage. Sorry to say it, but I see this a lot! I think that a pregnancy provides a perfect window for reintroducing some romance back into your relationship. Here is what I encourage you and your partner to do: sit down together and make a list of five things that you really enjoyed doing as a new couple. Then I encourage you to brainstorm five new activities you would like to add to the list. After you've completed your list of ten ideas, set aside time to do one of these activities each week. When couples make having fun and connecting with each other a priority, they grow closer as a couple. This list will also come in handy when you are getting through the early labor stage and looking for entertaining and distracting things to do before the birth.

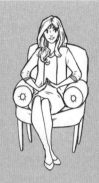
Another thing you can do is ask your partner to make a list of
ten things that makes him or her feel special and loved. This can be
anything from setting up the coffeepot in the morning to offering
a back rub to unexpectedly bringing home flowers. You get the
picture. Make the same list for your partner and then exchange
them. Commit to doing two things on your partner's list each
week, unannounced, no strings attached. You two are going to roll

up to the labor and delivery floor looking like two lovebirds. What better way to enter into co-parenting together, right?

UTILIZE EACH OTHER'S STRENGTHS

When you become a parent, and you are tired or cranky, it is easy to start harping on your partner's weaknesses. It is also easy to start playing the tit-for-tat game. Let me give you some examples of things I hear my clients saying to each other:

- I get up with the baby more than you, but you seem to be grumpier during the day.

- When was the last time you did a load of laundry around here?

- I always give you great back rubs. I can't remember the last time you massaged my shoulders.

- I feel like no one is helping me do the dishes or keep the house clean.

Instead of focusing on your partner's deficits or weaknesses, begin now with the practice of recognizing and celebrating strengths. Better yet, utilize and take advantage of each other's gifts. Your children will actually benefit if you are not exact clones of each other. One of you might be great at cooking while the other might be better at tidying up. You might love getting on the floor and playing with the kids; your partner might be really good at sleep training. Utilizing your unique strengths will serve you well, helping you to function as a team with your baby.

Not sure exactly what your or your partner's strengths are as they pertain to co-parenting? See the "Birth Guy's Strength Inventory" worksheet at http://www.newharbinger.com/41597. Download and print two copies. Circle your partner's strengths in one color, and yours in another. Ask your partner to do the same.

Then compare, contrast, and talk about how these strengths will come in handy after the baby has entered the picture.

ESTABLISH REGULAR CHECK-INS

Here is something that I notice quite a bit with the couples I work with: they might spend a lot of time in the same house or even the same workplace, but they usually don't *really spend time with each other*. Do you know what I mean by this? Couples often have smartphones in hand, or the TV blaring in the background. They're busy "doing life" and rushing past each other in the hallway. I encourage couples to put aside time weekly when they put down their phones, turn off the background noise, and *really* connect with each other. Ask your partner how she's doing. What were the highs and lows of her week? Does she have any concerns about your relationship or life in general? I know one couple that gets up half an hour early every day, grabs coffee, and has a little check-in before launching into their to-do list. This might not be possible for you, but I encourage you to find a regular time that you and your partner can check in with each other.

After the baby arrives, these check-ins will come in super handy. If Mom is home all day with the baby, she will really appreciate the face time she gets with you in the evening. Research shows that couples who make time for chitchat stay closer in the long run (Gottman and Silver 2000). And closer is really good when you are raising a baby, am I right?

Choosing Your Role Models Wisely

Let's talk a little about the people and voices that you and your partner surround yourselves with. Unlike the dads of the 1960s and 70s, who spent an average of ten to fifteen minutes with their little ones each day, the majority of modern-day dads and birth partners *want* to take a much more active role in the birth and parenting of their children. These days, it is not unusual for dads to care for their babies as much as, if not *more* than, moms. And yet, many of us are at a loss when trying to pinpoint positive role models due to the lack of parenting (or a surplus of negative parenting) that went down in our own childhoods. You might even feel anxiety about not having had a good role model growing up. *Am I going to suck as a parent? How am I going to know what to do?* The issue of role models was a big one for me when I was about to become a father, because my dad was not very present in my childhood.

Let me tell you that these doubts and concerns are totally normal. But there is something you can do about them. Surround yourself with positive role models now. Look around you…at work, in your friend group, in your family, and in your neighborhood. Identify the folks who you feel are doing the parenting thing well, and then meet with them and ask questions: What was the pregnancy and birth like for you? How did you support Mom through the experience? What do you love the most about being a parent? What suggestions do you have for me?

Because I didn't have a great relationship with my own father, I looked to several individuals in my life to serve as parenting examples and inspiration. Remember the family friend Bruce, whom I mentioned at the beginning of the book? He modeled for me how to be a present and involved dad, even when he was going through personal hardships. My Uncle Bill always took the time to call and check in with me. He pumped me full of confidence and showed me that life doesn't always have to be serious. He was a really jovial dude; I think I picked up my ability to always find fun with my kids from him. Uncle Bill also demonstrated what it is like to fully participate in parenting. The way he took an active role in raising his kids with his wife inspired me. My friends Luis and Joan were raising a baby when I was preparing to be a father. They were relaxed and seemed to really enjoy being parents, and they provided me with a template for what joyful co-parenting could look like. Finally, my best friend, Joey, was always cheering for me and being positive. He was the first visitor to hold my daughter Eva, and he is a loving and caring father today.

It is never too late to learn from mentors and to model yourself after them. This doesn't mean you'll get it perfect. None of us do, including your role models. We all stumble and fall, pick ourselves up, and learn as we go. But it helps a ton to have some rough guidelines in the form of other parents who are doing their best.

FOCUS ON POSITIVE OUTCOMES

Not only do you and your partner want to surround yourself with good people, you want to surround yourself with good messages. As a doula and birth educator, I hear a lot of negativity. Friends and family members don't mean any harm, but they tend to start telling doom-and-gloom stories the minute they find out your partner is pregnant.

I encourage you to create a "positive message agreement" with your partner. Agree that you will focus on positive stories and positive role models during the pregnancy. I promise you, there are five positive birth and parenting stories for every negative one, so seek out the positive ones. Surround yourself with couples and families who are approaching the task of parenthood with an adventurous and optimistic outlook. If a well-meaning friend or family member starts in with a horror story, politely let this person know that you prefer to hear about positive experiences because they give you something to aim for and they cause less anxiety.

In some ways, you and your partner get to shape your experiences of childbirth and parenting, so choose positive role models and messages while on this adventure. I'm not telling you to bury your head in the sand and pretend that pregnancy and parenting are always perfect experiences, because they aren't. I'm just encouraging you to focus your energy on what you *do want* instead of what you *don't*.

Counselor Corner: Establishing Strong Mental Health for You and Your Partner. Not only do you want to make sure that you go into the birth with your relationship in good shape, you want to make sure that both of you are feeling emotionally strong. Although postpartum depression has gained more attention in recent years, both in the medical field and the public eye, it is important to note that depression and anxiety can occur *during* a pregnancy as well. You might be surprised to hear this. You're supposed to be happy and excited 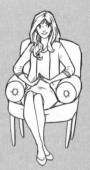 during a pregnancy, right? Well, sure...but not always. There are many factors that can contribute to depression or anxiety in pregnant moms:

- relationship challenges

- family or personal history of depression or anxiety

- infertility treatments that preceded the pregnancy

- previous pregnancy loss

- stressful life events

- complications during the pregnancy

- a history of abuse or trauma

Approximately 14 to 23 percent of women will struggle with some symptoms of depression during pregnancy, and many more will struggle with anxiety (Dietz et al. 2007). Professionals are beginning to use the term *perinatal mood and anxiety disorders*, or PMAD, to describe the emotional struggles or mental illness that women experience before, during, or after pregnancy. *Perinatal* means "before *and* after birth." Let's not leave out dads and birth partners, because they also might experience emotions that they didn't anticipate feeling before the baby arrives. Here are the common symptoms of depression to watch for:

- persistent sadness

- difficulty concentrating

- sleeping too little or too much

- loss of interest in activities that once brought joy

- recurring thoughts of death, suicide, or hopelessness

- anxiety (which can also be a stand-alone condition)

- feelings of guilt or worthlessness

- changes in eating habits

I share this information not to worry you, but to encourage you to seek help if you or Mom start exhibiting any of the above signs for more than two weeks. If so, start with Mom's ob-gyn or midwife, who can give you support and refer you to a counselor or psychiatrist if needed. Untreated depression in Mom during the pregnancy will lead to a higher likelihood of developing postpartum depression after the baby arrives, so it is important to seek treatment so Mom can feel prepared to handle the journey ahead. The good news is that depression and anxiety are highly treatable. If you seek help, things will most likely improve.

Maintaining Your Relationship for the Win!

Remember Taylor and Samantha from the beginning of the chapter? I'm happy to report that they are still together today and raising not one but two children. During my postpartum visits, I encouraged them to seek out support for their relationship. I also assigned many of the exercises we went over in this chapter. Taylor and Sam began to make their partnership a priority; they started to carve out a little bit of time each day to connect and check in with each other. With a counselor's help, Taylor took some time to explore his tendency to turn to alcohol when he was feeling stressed or overwhelmed. Sam also addressed her anxiety and explored ways to communicate her needs and concerns in a nonconfrontational manner. In the end, they rediscovered the reason that they fell in love in the first place and morphed into a powerful parenting pair. Creating lasting change in your relationship actually takes very little effort. If you follow the suggestions in this chapter you will definitely reap the romance benefits, both short-term and long-term.

BG FINAL SHOTS

✔ *Fortifying your relationship and addressing any unre-solved issues before childbirth is just as important as learning about breastfeeding or outfitting your nursery.* Your union with your partner came before the pregnancy, and it will hopefully be there long after your kiddo goes to college! Putting time and energy into strengthening your relationship will help you to be better parents and partners in the long run.

✔ *Use the nine to ten months of pregnancy to tune in to Mom's needs and court her as if you are dating again.* Turn on the music and slow dance. Bring home flowers unexpectedly. Spend as much time as you can chatting, reconnecting with each other, and having fun!

✔ *A pregnancy is a great time for extreme self-care.* Surround yourself with positive energy and role models. Address any mental health issues that come up for you or your partner. Just as you would tune up your car before a long road trip, this is a perfect time to tune up yourself and your relationship. You have some amazing adventures ahead—*make sure you fuel up for the journey!*

CHAPTER 3

Planning and Packing for the Birth

We've covered the basics and given your relationship a tune-up. Now it's time to start preparing for the birth! Let's begin by making a birth plan. If you don't know what a birth plan is, it is exactly what it sounds like: a rough game plan for how you and your partner would like the birth of your baby to unfold. Just as you make a plan when you go on vacation, you want to carefully think through how you want the birth of your child to go. Having a plan in place doesn't mean that things will go exactly as you want, but it *does* mean that you and your partner will feel more prepared and ready.

Some people caution that birth plans can create a false sense of security and that you won't be really sure how things are going to go, or how your partner is going to feel, until you are deep into the labor. You could argue the same thing about a vacation. There might be thunderstorms, you might get sick, or your rental car might break down. That doesn't mean that you can't create a rough blueprint for how you want your adventure to go and what you want to accomplish each day. It's the same with childbirth.

In my opinion, a birth plan helps you and your partner to clearly envision your ideal experience. It also helps you communicate your wishes and desires clearly with your birth professionals. The more that you plan out and imagine how you would like the experience to go, the more likely you are to have a positive experience. Of course, childbirth is always unpredictable. Sometimes you have to roll with the punches. But part of creating a plan is being prepared for those punches. Hang in there and I'll show you how.

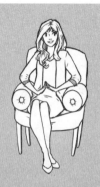
Before I share a few birth plans with you, I want to talk about five issues that will play into your plan: mobility, pushing, cord clamping and banking, breastfeeding, and rooming in. We're going to discuss these things in more detail in later chapters, but for now I want to give you an overview that will help you with your planning.

Mobility

Let's discuss how much Mom wants to move around during labor. If she says, "I want an epidural ordered up as soon as I get to the hospital," that is completely okay. But if she says, "I would really like to have a natural childbirth, with as little intervention as possible," then we need to talk about mobility. Doing squats, bouncing on an exercise ball, walking around the room, and changing positions can all help move labor in the right direction. I call it "laboring down"—helping the baby to move down the birth canal. Mom might want to deliver the baby on her knees or in a squatting position. If this is the case, there are requests of the hospital staff you will want to make to increase Mom's mobility.

THREE MOBILITY CRUSHERS

There are three standard hospital interventions that can impact mobility: epidurals, IVs, and fetal heart-rate monitoring. Being fully informed about these common practices can help you and Mom put together your birth plan.

Epidural anesthesia is a numbing medicine that is injected into the space around the spinal nerves in the lower back. It numbs the area above and below the point of injection and allows Mom to remain awake during delivery. If administered correctly, it relieves Mom of all pain from labor contractions. It can be used for either a vaginal birth or a cesarean delivery. A doctor who is an anesthesia specialist administers the epidural anesthesia. When Mom has an epidural, pain is subtracted from the equation, but so is mobility.

Intravenous therapy, commonly known as an IV, is the infusion of liquid substances directly into a vein, usually in a hand or an arm. The intravenous route is the fastest way to deliver fluids and medications throughout the body. Hospital staff usually connect Mom to an IV when she checks into her hospital room in case fluids, antibiotics, or other medicines need to be administered during labor. You can imagine that being connected to an IV stand, even if it is on wheels, is going to mess with Mom's ability to move around. If Mom is aiming for maximum mobility, request that a saline lock (commonly referred to as a hep-lock) be used. This small port is attached to her hand and can be connected to an IV if needed.

Fetal heart-rate monitoring is the process of checking the condition of the baby during labor and delivery by monitoring his or her heart rate. There are a few different ways to do this. One method involves connecting Mom, via wires, to monitoring equipment that is usually near the hospital bed. However, if you're going for more mobility and movement, you can request intermittent or wireless monitoring.

You are probably beginning to notice a theme. There are a lot of contraptions that might be attached to Mom in the hospital. I like to use different types of computers to illustrate her potential experience. Consider a desktop computer versus a laptop. A laptop is untethered. You can carry it to a coffee shop, the park, or a kitchen table, and work wherever you want. The downside is that it is not connected to a power source, so you have to periodically plug it in. A desktop computer is continually plugged in and receiving power, but it cannot be moved without great effort. In the hospital room, if Mom has an epidural and all of the various devices are connected to her body, there is a constant flow of data and fluids, but her mobility will be limited.

There is no wrong or right—it is just good to know your options and to be prepared to talk to your nurses and health care providers about them. Let's review mobility using the table below.

Mobility Review

More Mobile	Less Mobile
Intermittent or wireless fetal heart-rate monitoring	Wired fetal heart-rate monitoring
Hep-lock/saline lock (a small port that can be connected to an IV if needed)	IV (a device that allows fluid to flow directly into a patient's veins)
No epidural	Epidural

One last note about mobility: Even if Mom wants maximum movement and mobility, the nurses will still need to occasionally plug her in and make sure the baby is doing okay. This is just the way things are done at the hospital, so please don't get angry at the nurses. They're just doing their thing.

TO EPIDURAL OR NOT TO EPIDURAL

It is important to understand and respect Mom's wishes when it comes to pain relief and interventions, and to not judge. Everyone has a different tolerance for pain, and everyone has been through different experiences in life. Sometimes these experiences were traumatic. It's important to keep in mind that you and your partner are bringing a baby into the world—and that is exciting stuff, regardless of how the delivery unfolds.

If Mom says, "I want an epidural as soon as I walk in the room," let the nurse know and look forward to possibly taking a little nap or watching a movie during the labor.

If Mom says, "Let's try to do the birth without an epidural," this is an important thing to note. Nurses will frequently say to Mom, "Let me know when you are ready for an epidural," or "Are you ready for some relief from that pain?" Feel free to say to the staff, "Please don't ask us about pain meds. We will ask you if Mom wants or needs them." This will allow you and Mom to determine how and when pain relief is administered.

When I think of epidurals, I think of Kris and Tom, a couple who attended my birth class, Facilitating Fearless Birth, and then hired me as their doula to attend their hospital birth. When we were cocreating their birth plan, Tom encouraged Kris to try for a medication-free birth. He felt like Kris would be a "rock star" and promised her that he would coach her through the experience. Kris wasn't so sure. She admitted to me that she didn't have a great tolerance for pain. As we talked more, Kris shared that she was abused as a child. "I've done a lot of counseling and healing over the years, but I'm still not a big fan of pain and trauma, if you know what I mean."

I assured Kris that I *did* know what she meant. The three of us talked some more, and Kris decided that she would go into the hospital with a plan to have an intervention-free birth. However, Kris and Tom also agreed that if Kris gave the word, they'd request an epidural, no questions asked.

When Kris went into active labor and we met up at the hospital, Tom requested a hep-lock and intermittent monitoring, as they had laid out in their birth plan, so that Kris could move around. And move around she did! She bounced on an exercise ball. She and Tom used a rebozo scarf (which I will discuss in more detail later). She squatted in a warm bath for a bit. Kris really helped that baby to start moving down the birth canal. After laboring for a few hours, she turned to Tom and said, "Okay, honey. I'm ready for that epidural. Get on it." Tom grabbed a nurse, requested the epidural, and we all got to rest for several hours before she began pushing. I loved seeing this couple support each other and communicate openly, before and during their labor.

Pushing

Let's talk about that last part of labor that gets your baby out into the world. When I say pushing, I'm not just talking about the precise moment when Mom pushes the baby out. I'm actually talking about the space of time from when Mom begins to push to when the baby actually appears.

For a first birth, pushing can last forty-five minutes to more than two hours. On TV and in the movies, they make this process seem loud, quick, and easy, but it can actually take quite a while.

There are a few things that can make pushing easier. Most midwives will let Mom push in a squatting position or on her hands and knees when at home or in a birth center. Gravity and the opening of the birth canal in these positions can really help that baby come into the world. However, in a hospital, depending on the circumstances, it is likely that Mom will be directed to push while lying on her back. In this position, her sacrum comes up and the baby has to get over a hump. This makes pushing a little more challenging. Millions of women give birth this way every year, but if your doctor or hospital is open to pushing in different positions, you might want to have that discussion with both Mom and your nurse. Mom might also want to try following her instincts and direct her own pushing instead of being directed. Discuss these things with your doctor beforehand, and then mark them on your plan.

Cord Clamping and Banking

The *umbilical cord* is the thick ropelike tube that connects an opening in the baby's stomach to the placenta in the womb. The average cord is about 20 inches long. It carries oxygen and nutrients—needed to keep the baby alive during the pregnancy— from the placenta to your baby's bloodstream. Soon after the birth, the cord will be clamped 1½ to 2 inches from baby's belly button with a plastic clip. Your doctor or midwife will place another clamp at the other end of the cord, near the placenta, and then cut the cord between the two clamps, leaving a stump about 1 to 1½ inches long on your baby's tummy. This will form the belly button when it's healed. Amazing, right?

More and more doctors and birth professionals are recommending delaying clamping and cord cutting. They argue that good nutrients and blood will continue flowing into the baby as he or she adjusts to being in the outside world. I bring this issue up because these are good things to ask your doctor about, decide on, and put in your birth plan. Can Dad cut the cord? Can we delay cutting and clamping the cord? What does that process look like, and how long can we delay it? If you decide to bank your baby's stem cells, however, delaying the clamping and cutting might not be an option.

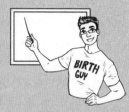

Birth Guy Pointer: Consider Banking Cord Blood and Placental Cells. When my two babies were born more than a decade ago, we didn't invest in cord-blood banking. This process involves collecting blood stem cells directly after the birth and storing them for future medical use by your family. At the time, we didn't feel like there was enough evidence to justify the investment. Fast-forward to 2015, when my oldest daughter was diagnosed with Lyme disease. After much research on treatment options, we opted for an infusion treatment that included stem cell transplantation. If we had banked my daughter's cells, this treatment, which really saved my daughter's health, would have been less expensive and more accessible. This was an eye-opening experience for me.

LifebankUSA is doing incredible research with both cord blood *and* placental blood. Led by Dr. Hariri, a neurosurgeon, the company is currently conducting clinical research on how placental stem cells can be used to treat various diseases, such as acute myeloid leukemia, Crohn's disease, diabetic peripheral neuropathy, and diabetic foot ulcers. The research the company is performing and the banking options it provides are groundbreaking and game-changing. I encourage you to contact LifebankUSA if you want to learn more about what is involved with banking your baby's stem cells.

Optimizing Breastfeeding Conditions

You will see a few items on the birth plan that refer to formula, pacifiers, and cup feeding. I'm not going into great detail on breastfeeding in this section because I devoted all of chapter 8 to the topic. If you and Mom plan on attempting breastfeeding, you will want to avoid things in the hospital such as bottles, formula, and pacifiers, which might hinder Mom and your baby's progress with breastfeeding technique and flow. For instance, if the hospital determines that formula is necessary for your newborn, it is preferable that staff give the formula through a syringe so your baby doesn't get accustomed to a bottle nipple. I suggest that you review chapter 8 prior to making your birth plan. That chapter will help you to set up an ideal environment for breastfeeding success.

Rooming In

"Rooming in" has a cool sound to it, huh? It means that your baby stays in the hospital room with you and Mom. You know those TV shows and cartoons that show all the babies lined up in little bassinets in a hospital nursery, and the parents look through a window for the baby with the correct name tag? And they hope their baby doesn't get mixed up with another one? Ha, ha! Well, those days are becoming a thing of the past. Hospitals are becoming more open to and encouraging of the baby sleeping in the same room with Mom and Dad. This way, Mom and the baby are never separated, and she can respond to the baby's needs immediately. More skin-to-skin contact and natural bonding are the results of rooming in. And a bonus is that Dad is available and ready to help when Mom needs a breather. Some hospitals still have nurseries where the baby can stay if Mom and Dad need a break. If you would prefer the baby to stay in your room the entire time you're at the hospital, let the nurses know on your birth plan.

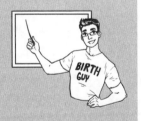

Birth Guy Pointer: Come Bearing Gifts for the Staff. As you can see, there are several requests you are going to be making of the hospital staff to help the birth go as planned. It's a great idea to show them your appreciation with snacks or treats. Send a friend or family member out for donuts or muffins. Let the nurses know how much you appreciate them partnering with you and Mom. Let's get this team off on the right foot! You have some amazing work to do together.

Birth Plan Templates

If you do an online search, you can typically find premade birth plan templates. However, they tend to be a bit lengthy. Truth be told, I've witnessed labor and delivery nurses rolling their eyes at five-page plans. Most birth professionals whom I encounter like parents to keep the plan succinct and simple. For this reason, I created the following birth plans, both available for download at http://www.newharbinger.com/41597. Birth plan #1 is designed for parents who are aiming for more mobility, an unmedicated childbirth, and optimized conditions for breastfeeding. Birth plan #2 is designed for parents who are open to an epidural or formula feeding, or both.

Birth Guy's Birth Plan #1

Thank you for helping our family deliver our new baby. We appreciate your time looking over our plan and helping us achieve our goals.

→ We would prefer a hep-lock versus an IV connected to a pump.

→ We would like intermittent or wireless monitoring for maximum mobility, if possible.

→ Please do not ask us if we want pain medicine or an epidural. We will ask you if it becomes necessary.

→ Mom prefers to push while squatting or on hands and knees.

→ Directed pushing is okay, but Mom can self-direct if circumstances are right.

→ Dad would like to cut the cord. We would also like delayed cord clamping and cord banking.

- ➔ We would like immediate skin-to-skin contact for Mom and the baby.

- ➔ No pacifiers or bottles, please.

- ➔ No formula, if possible. IF formula is needed, please feed with a syringe ONLY.

- ➔ Rooming in with the baby, please.

Birth Guy's Birth Plan #2

Thank you for helping our family deliver our new baby. We appreciate your time looking over our plan and helping us achieve our goals.

- ➔ We would like an epidural as soon as Mom feels pain.

- ➔ We understand that this will decrease mobility for Mom.

- ➔ Directed pushing is fine.

- ➔ Dad would like to cut the cord. We would also like delayed cord clamping and cord banking.

- ➔ We would like immediate skin-to-skin contact for Mom and the baby.

- ➔ We will attempt to breastfeed, but formula is okay.

- ➔ Rooming in with baby is preferred, but nursery time is okay.

As you look through these birth plans, you might be wondering why there isn't a plan involving cesarean sections. I cover C-sections and other birth situations in great detail in chapter 7, where I'll give you pointers on how to have a positive C-section experience. Stay tuned for that info, because I definitely want to prepare you for these potential experiences.

Creating Your Personal Birth Plan

The birth plan templates provided on the previous pages are designed for you and your partner to give to a nurse at the hospital. As I've already explained, you want to keep your birth plan fairly simple and focused on medical interventions. In this section, I'm going to talk about making a personal plan for your hospital (or birth center) stay. This plan involves the more intimate parts of your experience and will help you to create an environment that feels comfortable and safe. The personal plan stays between you and your partner. Here are some questions to help you create a personal birth plan:

- If Mom's water breaks and you have to leave suddenly for the hospital, are there neighbors or family members who can care for your house, other children, or your pets?

- What kind of music do you want to listen to in the labor room? How do you want to listen to it?

- Who do you want in the room during labor? During the birth? Following the birth? While Mom is breastfeeding?

- Is it okay for the birth to be photographed or recorded on video? Who will operate the camera?

- Do you have a code word for when the pain gets intense and Mom wants Dad to try another labor technique or request an epidural? How about a code word for when Mom is feeling crowded by visitors and wants to clear the room so she can get some rest or breastfeed in peace?

- How are you going to handle social media? Who gets to make the first post about the birth? Does Mom want to approve any photos before they're posted? (I'm guessing the answer is "hell, yes!")

- Is Dad going to sleep in the room? If so, what will he need to sleep comfortably?

- Are there take-out restaurants near the hospital that you like? (Dad might need to order food in, or have a friend bring food, so have take-out menus handy.)

- If you have a little dude, do you want him circumcised? Do you want it to happen in the hospital or at a later date?

- Which car do you want to travel to and from the hospital in? Will it accommodate a car seat? (You will need to have that bad boy hooked up and ready to go.)

The "Birth Guy's Personal Birth Plan" worksheet, available for download at http://www.newharbinger.com/41597, can help you work through these questions. Having filled it out with your partner will make your hospital stay feel more comfortable and customized.

Taking a Hospital Tour Before Labor

I encourage all of my clients to arrange a tour during their second or third trimester. A hospital or birth center tour is similar to a "meet the teacher" night. Instead of the classroom, you're scoping out the delivery room. Instead of meeting your teacher, you're meeting the staff. You and Mom will feel so much more prepared for the birth of your baby if you know exactly where to go and what to expect when you arrive at the hospital. A scheduled visit offers you a great opportunity to ask the staff questions and make sure that the facility is a match for your birth plans and philosophy. Below are some things to investigate during your tour. Many of these questions are geared toward a large hospital, but they can apply to a birth center as well:

- What is the parking situation like? Are there spots designated for parents in labor?

- Where is the entrance for the labor and delivery ward? Where do you check in when you arrive at the hospital? What are the check-in procedures?

- Can you preregister for the birth so you have minimal paperwork and check-in questions when you arrive?

- Do the staff seem warm and friendly? Do they seem to like their jobs? (Chat with them.)

- What kind of labor tools are provided? Peanut balls or yoga balls? (The more stuff that the hospital provides, the less you need to tote along with you.)

- Are there bathtubs in the delivery rooms? Do moms get to be in the bath at any point during the delivery?

- Does the staff encourage mobility? Is a hep-lock offered instead of an IV? Wireless monitoring instead of wired monitoring? Are squat bars and other aids for pushing in different positions provided? (Remember that birth plan, guys? Bring it along with you for reference.)

- How is the labor and delivery ward divided? Are there separate rooms for triage, labor and delivery, and recovery? Is there a nursery? (Ask to see all of the spaces that are available.)

- What is the policy for visitors? Are there visiting hours? Does the hospital partner with doulas? If so, when does staff recommend that the doula arrive?

- What is the food situation? Does Dad get meals or does he need to order out? Are there vending machines available for light snacking?

Most of these questions will be answered as standard protocol during your tour. However, I want you to have them in mind in case there are any gaps in the information provided.

Packing for the Hospital or Birth Center

Okay, you've planned for the birth, similar to planning for a vacation. You've previewed the place you'll be staying at (that is, the hospital or birth center). Now it's time to pack your suitcase for the birth adventure. Think of this as a staycation at the hospital. That puts a cool spin on things, right?

Typically, a few weeks before her due date, Mom packs a bag, which includes a nightgown, a cute outfit for the baby, maybe a special pillow, and some toiletries. If you are planning to have your baby at a birth center or at home, your midwife will give Mom a list of items to purchase for a "birth kit." If you're heading to a hospital, staff will provide a lot of medical supplies but not a lot of labor or comfort supplies. You usually have to bring this stuff with you.

I like to involve dads and birth partners in this part of the preparation. You'll be Mom's coach, personal assistant, and counselor for a few days, so you'll want some tools to help her have a positive birth and postbirth experience. I'll also note that you will be spending just as much time at the hospital as Mom, so you might want some creature comforts of your own.

ITEMS TO BRING TO THE HOSPITAL

The hours I have spent in hospital rooms are probably too many to count. I've become intimately familiar with the inner workings of these sometimes sterile and utilitarian rooms. Throughout the years, I've identified many items—Birth Guy must-haves—that Dad can bring to warm up the space and to make labor more comfortable.

Twin-size blanket: Aim for a comfy and cozy little blanket. Go for a darker color, because hospital colors are usually neutral and drab. Tossing a dark or brightly colored blanket over the bed or a chair can add some energy to the room and provide Mom with soft comfort and warmth later.

Essential oils: Okay, I'm not an essential-oil expert, but I will tell you that natural aromatic oils are the bomb. Lavender and peppermint are fantastic ones to start with. Lavender generally makes people feel comforted and at ease. It also gives you that spa-like feeling. Let's be honest, hospitals don't smell great, so the scent of lavender can be a great addition to the room. Peppermint can help Mom if she is experiencing nausea during labor. Here's a fun idea: take Mom with you to a health-food store during the pregnancy to sniff the various oils and pick out her favorites. Can you feel those brownie points adding up, guys?

Birth Guy Pointer: Using the Supplies in Your Hospital Room. Check out the hospital room when you arrive. Look in all of the drawers and closets and see what you have available. Usually you will find some clean folded towels. Pull out a few little ones and place them by the sink. When Mom is feeling nauseated, you can put a touch of peppermint oil and some cold water on one and wrap it around Mom's neck. This will cool her off and give her some relief from the nausea.

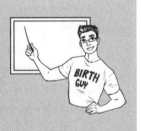

Acupressure wristbands: For twenty-three centuries, acupressure has been used to treat and alleviate physical symptoms in humans. That's a long time, right? According to acupuncture and acupressure practitioners, applying gentle pressure to the P6 (or nei-kuan)

acupressure point on your wrists can alleviate nausea. You can apply this pressure manually (see the graphic below), or you can purchase wristbands that will apply it for you. Many people swear that these bracelets help them with nausea and seasickness. It is common for moms to experience nausea during labor, so it's a great idea to have a couple of these bracelets handy. You can purchase them online or at most drugstores.

The P6 Acupressure Point

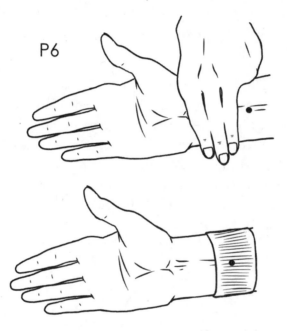

Hot water bottle: Do you remember old-school hot water bottles from your childhood that look like a big rubber bladder? You can buy them at a drugstore or online. When Mom's back starts to hurt during labor, you can fill one of these bad boys with hot water and apply it to the small of Mom's back. It's incredible what a difference a little bit of heat makes. Quick and easy relief!

Exercise ball: Okay, guys, this is a big must-have. Mom can gently rock or bounce on the ball or drape herself over it for laboring down, as I discussed earlier. Look for a weighted exercise ball with sand in it. These stay put and are less likely to roll around the room. Mom will also be less likely to lose her balance and roll off. This ball will be a lifesaver during labor, helping her stay mobile and moving that baby down the birth canal.

Yoga mats: If Mom wants to try for an unmedicated birth, or try to labor it out for a while without meds, you can put one or two yoga mats down so Mom can sit on the floor or get on her hands and knees. With the mats in place, neither of you will be grossed-out by whatever floor you're on.

Peanut ball: This inflatable rubber ball that looks like a peanut will be super helpful if Mom is laboring in bed or has had an epidural. Blow it up to three-quarters of its capacity, not all the way, and place it between Mom's legs while she is lying on her side. You can also push the ball up against the base of Mom's pelvis a little, which will help open things up and move the baby down. Your nurse or doula can help you with the placement.

Peanut Ball

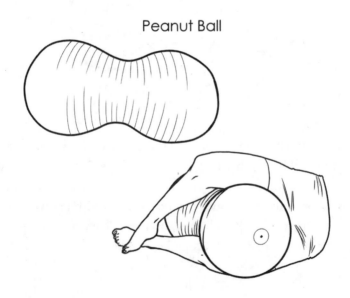

Rebozo scarf: This long scarf, which you can easily find online, is one of my favorite tools to use with couples when Mom is working through active labor. You can also view a video on "Rebozo Techniques for Active Labor" at http://www.newharbinger. com/41597 that will show you how to use the scarf. Choose Mom's favorite color so she can use it as a nursing wrap or shawl later on. I'm all about repurposing!

Music: Back when I attended my first births, you had to lug a massive boom box into the labor room if you wanted tunes. Those days are behind us now that we have so many music-streaming options. Chat with Mom about what kind of music she wants to listen to. This is a great opportunity to collaborate on the mood and feel that you both want in the room.

Bag o' technology: You brought music. Now you need technology to broadcast it. Prepare a bag full of everything you need to be fully wired in your hospital room. Remember that you might be staying at the hospital for two to three days, or even longer, depending on the circumstances. So, think about all of the gadgets that will help you to stay connected. Here's the list I usually give to dads:

- Wireless speaker

- Smartphones (Well, duh, right? But you would be surprised how many couples forget their phones when flying out the door to the hospital.)

- Laptop or tablet, or both

- Chargers for your phones, laptop, tablet, and speaker

- Camera

I also recommend that you throw in a couple of extension cords. The available outlets might be clear across the room from Mom's bed, and she might want to reach her charging phone while breastfeeding.

Push present: Occasionally, one of my dads will give his partner a sweet gift when she goes into labor or following the birth. Affectionately called a "push present," the gift is designed to give Mom a little extra encouragement for the hard work she is about to do or gratitude for the work she's done. These gifts can range from expensive jewelry to a cute T-shirt to a sweet poem or note. They are not really necessary, or expected by most moms, but they can definitely be a sweet touch after Mom has worked her butt off!

Car seat: I've mentioned the car seat a few times, but I'm going to mention it again. You need a safe way to bring your little bundle of love home. I recommend that you purchase an infant car seat at least one month before the due date. Read the directions or, better yet, get some assistance from a certified car-seat expert. Car seats can be tricky to install the first time. Take your time, and then practice getting it in and out of the car a few times. You will be happy that you did so when it is time to load up junior.

> *I partnered with Winston and Tanisha before, during, and after the birth of their daughter. I met Winston during one of my Rocking Dads classes. He was one of those dads who listened to every word I said and took full pages of notes—love this guy! When I met the couple at the hospital, Winston had his arms completely full. Yoga mat under one arm, weighted ball under the other, and a bag o' technology slung over his shoulder. The nurses oohed and aahed over his supplies. He continued to impress as he traded out his tools in the labor room, responding to Tanisha's needs every step of the way. One minute he was using the rebozo scarf, the next he was helping Tanisha balance on the exercise ball. He had a cool peppermint-scented towel ready for her neck and a hot water bottle for her back. Ella Fitzgerald was playing in the background when their baby girl was delivered vaginally. Watching Winston in action was inspiring. I have to admit, I was a proud doula in that moment. Watching him give Tanisha a sweet charm bracelet after the birth and seeing her emotional appreciation for Winston's efforts made me tear up.*

When I swung by the hospital two mornings later for a quick postpartum visit, we debriefed the birth and talked about preparing to go home. That's when Winston realized that he had forgotten the car seat at the house. No biggie. Even the most prepared dads forget things sometimes. I stayed with Tanisha and helped her work on breastfeeding while Winston ran home and installed the car seat. He was back within an hour and ready to drive his little family home.

Mom Moment: Mom's Bag of Goodies. Mom really doesn't need much for a birth. As long as she brings her body, the hospital or birth center will take care of the rest. Nevertheless, here are a few of the items that I've found can really improve Mom's hospital or birth center experience:

- *A nightgown:* A hospital gown will work fine, but if Mom wants to wear something a little more visually appealing, she should bring her own. Make sure it isn't too long, or else it will get tangled up during the labor and delivery, and it should have buttons or snaps in the front for breastfeeding and skin-to-skin access. It also helps if it has easy access in the back in case Mom wants or needs an epidural. Since you will be in the hospital for a few days, Mom will want to pack a few different comfy lounging outfits, all with easy access for breastfeeding.

- *Facial wipes:* If Mom arrives at the hospital in full makeup, it might be a while before she can get to the sink to wash it off. Let me tell you, there is nothing like labor to smear that mascara all over the place. Facial wipes can be used to remove makeup, sweat, *and* tears. The best thing is, Mom doesn't have to get out of bed to use them.

- *Hair ties:* I'm a girl of the 1990s, so I'm still partial to scrunchies. Embarrassing but true. It doesn't matter what Mom uses to tie her hair back, but she will definitely want something. Being in labor is sort of like combining a dance contest with a marathon with a roller coaster. Let's keep that hair out of the way so Mom can focus on the hard work ahead of her.

- *Flip-flops:* Everyone recommends slippers. Slippers are nice, but, as their name implies, they can be slippery. Flip-flops are easy to slide feet into and can be worn in the bathroom or the shower.

- *Toilet paper:* This might sound silly, but the toilet paper in a hospital can be a little rough, and Mom's rear end is going be a little raw. One roll of soft toilet paper from home might just be a lifesaver for Mom.

- *Granny panties:* The hospital will give Mom some large mesh undies to hold superlarge pads. If Mom wants to forgo the mesh, she can bring her own large underwear.

- *Earplugs and an eye mask:* Anyone who has been in a hospital room knows that they are not the most quiet or dark places. If Mom has difficulty sleeping in strange places, she might want to bring a few sleep aids to help out.

- *Different size outfits for the baby:* We're not sure how big that baby is going to be until he or she comes out, so pack a newborn and a three-month-size outfit. Throw in soft little socks and a baby hat to keep your little one warm on the way home.

- *Baby book:* If you already have a book to document your baby's first year, bring it along to the hospital. Dad can write in a few of the stats and details in real time. A nurse will also ink up your sweet baby's feet and make little prints in the book.

- *An extra bag:* You'll be gifted with a lot of extra goodies at the hospital. Baby blankets, paperwork, mesh undies, and big absorbent pads, not to mention the sweet gifts from visitors. Bring along an extra bag to tote it all home.

WHAT ABOUT THE KITCHEN SINK?

You might feel like I am asking you to pack your entire house for this birth. I know it seems like a lot. If you lay out the items listed in this chapter on your bed, however, they really don't add up to that much. That being said, pick and choose the items that feel important and helpful to you. Remember that the hospital or the birth center will have the essentials that you need to have a safe and memorable birth. You can always send a family member or friend to the house if you realize you forgot something. You're not traveling to another country, just to a brand-new chapter in your life!

BG FINAL SHOTS

✔ *Making a birth plan not only helps you to clearly communicate your wants and needs to your medical team, it also helps you and Mom to start envisioning and manifesting a positive birth experience.* Keep it simple, have some fun, and reach out to a birth professional for help if needed.

✔ *When Dad purchases and packs items for the hospital, he lets Mom know that he is fully prepared and pumped for the birth.* Go through the lists and select the items that feel the most helpful to both of you.

✔ *The most important things you need for this birth are you, Mom, and a great attitude.* Don't be shocked if things go a little off course with your birth plan. Don't worry if something gets accidentally left at home or unpurchased. In the end, you will be holding a beautiful baby. Everything else will fade in comparison.

CHAPTER 4

Navigating Early Labor at Home

I first met Lamar and Tonya at one of my ultrasound clinics. Their enthusiasm was unforgettable—I almost had to cover my ears at one point because they were crying and cheering so loudly in the imaging room. They hired me as their doula and attended various classes of mine, bringing their contagious enthusiasm with them every step of the way.

One early Wednesday morning, two days from Tonya's due date, I received a phone call. "BRIAN!!! I think Tonya is in labor! Should we go to the hospital? Should I call an ambulance?" Lamar yelled into the phone. In the background, I could hear shrieking.

"Lamar, take a breath, buddy," I urged. "Give me some information before we make any decisions. How many contractions has Tonya had? Has her water broken? Give me the scoop."

"I think this is her second contraction. She had one about fifteen minutes ago. We weren't sure what it was. She said it felt like a really strong cramp. Now we're on to number two. Pretty sure she's in labor, man. No water or anything leaking yet. What do I do, Brian? This is crazy, huh? Wow! I'm going to be a Dad!" Lamar was talking so fast I could barely catch what he was saying.

"Yup, you're definitely going to be a Dad soon, but not quite yet," I explained. "Sounds like Tonya is in early labor. With

contractions that far apart, it's probably going to be a little while before we head to the hospital. Take some deep breaths, Lamar. Time to pull out those Jedi-like skills we talked about. Your job is to help Tonya stay calm and comfortable while she works through this initial part of the labor. You're going to do fine, Lamar. You're going to be amazing!"

Lamar and Tonya's story is not unusual. Their exuberance is a little unusual…but not their preconceived beliefs about labor. Thanks to movies and TV, many people think that the minute a woman goes into labor, it's important to put her in the car and get her to the hospital.

The truth is that for *most* couples, a large portion of the labor will happen at home. As long as Mom doesn't have any preexisting conditions or pregnancy complications, the hospital will probably not want to see you until Mom's cervix is dilated to five or six centimeters and her contractions are five or fewer minutes apart. This can take a long time—anywhere from several weeks to a few hours. In Lamar and Tonya's case, it took about ten hours. By 8 p.m. that evening, Tonya's contractions were coming every five minutes. We had her settled in the hospital room by 9:30 p.m.

I'm going to give you plenty of hints for how to soothe Mom and make her comfortable while you stay at home and prepare for active labor. But before I do that, I want to define some terms that you will need to know as you move through the next few chapters.

Labor Vocabulary

When I meet with an expectant couple, I try not to flood them with loads of medical or technical jargon. They're usually not going for a medical degree, they're just trying to understand how pregnancy and childbirth work. Below are a few terms that are key to the labor and delivery experience. Feel free to ask your provider for more details if you want to dive deeper into the terminology.

Cervix: The cylinder-shaped neck of tissue that connects the vagina and the uterus, or womb. Think of this as the exit door for your baby.

Dilation: The widening and opening of the cervix, measured in centimeters. The cervix will go from zero to ten centimeters in diameter and have a width similar to that of a bagel when completely dilated. Mom's cervix prepares for delivery by providing an opening from the uterus to the birth canal, unblocking your baby's exit route. Early labor opens the exit up to about six centimeters. Active labor opens things up to ten centimeters.

Contractions: The periodic tightening and relaxing of the uterine muscle, the largest muscle in a woman's body, which helps the cervix to open up. Contractions can range from mild period-like cramping sensations (early, early labor) to crazy, intense sensations (later labor). The uterine muscle has a lot of work to do to open that exit door for the baby. There's a reason they call it labor and not vacation.

Prelabor: Occurring one to four weeks before labor begins, it's the period of time when Mom will start to notice changes in her body as it prepares for the birth. In the next section, I'm going to give you the lowdown on which changes to look for and how Mom might be affected.

Early labor: The period of time from the onset of labor until the cervix has dilated to six centimeters. This can begin weeks before the birth or it might start eight hours before the birth. It definitely varies from woman to woman and pregnancy to pregnancy.

Active labor: This phase of labor is pretty intense and usually lasts a few hours, although there is a wide range of what is considered normal. I'll give you the full scoop on active labor, and how to support your partner through the experience, in chapter 5.

Keep this vocabulary in mind as we move forward. You're going to hear these terms *a lot* as I teach you all about labor and delivery. Before we launch into my tools and tips for early labor, let's talk about the signs that let you know labor is on the horizon.

Prelabor—Mom's Body Is Getting Ready

One to four weeks before Mom goes into early labor, her body starts prepping for the big day, similar to the way a football team gears up during preseason. At this point in the pregnancy, you and Mom will probably be going to weekly prenatal appointments. Mom's provider will be on the lookout for the following common indicators that the baby will be making an appearance soon.

Baby begins to drop. A few weeks before labor begins, the baby might start descending in Mom's pelvis. This is also referred to as "lightening," which is humorous, because Mom will feel anything but light. She will most likely feel more pressure and weight as the baby moves into the birth position: head down and low. Mom will be waddling more than ever and making plenty of trips to the bathroom. The baby will be putting major pressure on her bladder.

Mom's cervix begins to dilate. As we discussed earlier, the cervix has a lot of work to do in order to open the exit for the baby. It might begin doing this work weeks before labor even begins. Your provider will check the cervix for dilating (opening) and effacing (thinning out) during weekly appointments. Don't be disappointed if Mom's cervix is dilating slowly. Everyone progresses at their own speed.

She feels more cramps and increased back pain. Everything in Mom's body is shifting and stretching in preparation for birth. In addition, she has a baby the size of a basketball in her abdomen. That's a lot of weight out front! Some discomfort is to be expected.

Her joints feel like they are loosening. The hormone relaxin helps to soften and loosen all of Mom's ligaments. Some people say that this loosening effect causes Mom to be a bit clumsy in the last trimester. Encourage her to exercise extra caution as she moves through these last few weeks.

She complains about diarrhea. Her joints aren't the only things that are loosening. Muscles are also starting to relax, including the rectum, which can lead to loose bowel movements. Remind Mom to stay hydrated and reassure her that this is a good sign!

She wakes up more frequently during the night. Mom might start waking up every two to three hours to use the restroom. Don't be surprised if she is waking you up as well. I believe that this is nature's way of preparing the two of you to be parents and to get ready for those night feedings.

She loses her mucus plug. A mucus plug is exactly what it sounds like: a gooey, gelatinous plug that blocks the cervical canal and protects the uterus from bacteria and pathogens. When Mom's cervix starts to open up, her mucus plug might release and fall out. The plug is usually off-white in color with streaks of pink, like something that came out of your nose. This is kind of gross, but true. Loss of the mucus plug means that labor will most likely start within the next two to three weeks, sometimes sooner.

She experiences Braxton Hicks contractions. These painless and irregular contractions are named for John Braxton Hicks, the English doctor who first described them in 1872. Moms usually describe these contractions as a feeling of tightening and then relaxing in their uterus or lower abdominal area.

If any of the above changes are happening, then Mom's body is preparing for the big day. The only challenge is that we don't know how long this preseason will last. It could be days before labor starts, or weeks. Reassure Mom that her body knows what to do and that labor will start when the timing is right.

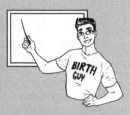
When Prelabor Transitions to Early Labor

The questions I hear the most in my Rocking Dads classes are:
How will I know if Mom is in labor? What should I be looking for?
I explain that the timing of Mom's contractions is everything. Her
contractions should be no more than twenty minutes apart and no
less than five minutes apart. If the contractions are more than
twenty minutes apart, Mom isn't in actual labor. She might be
experiencing Braxton Hicks contractions, or practice contractions.
These are the body's warm-up exercises for the birth, and they
might start weeks before the birth.

If the contractions are fewer than five minutes apart, Mom is
moving into active labor and should be heading to the hospital.
The baby is most likely on the way. I encourage all of my clients to
ask their health care provider two questions during their third-
trimester appointments:

1. At what point in Mom's labor should we call you (or the office)?

2. When should we head to the hospital (or birth center)?

If Mom has a preexisting condition or a pregnancy complication, her doctor, and possibly a fetal-maternal medical specialist, will determine when she should go to the hospital and what kind of care she will receive. However, if Mom is experiencing a healthy, normal pregnancy, her provider will probably encourage her to "labor it out" at home until she goes into active labor.

Always trust your gut. On rare occasions, early labor speeds ahead quickly and Mom is ready for go time within a few hours. I will talk more about this and other circumstances at the end of the chapter. Don't be afraid or embarrassed to call your doctor (even if it is the middle of the night) if things are getting intense. Your provider gets many of these calls and is prepared to answer any questions you might have. I provided a handy chart below to help you keep in mind the stages of labor.

Stages of Labor Review: From Prelabor Through Active Labor

Length of Time Between Contractions	Stage of Labor
More than twenty minutes apart	Prelabor *Mom's body is warming up for labor.*
Between five and twenty minutes apart	Early labor *Most of the time, couples are directed to work through early labor at home.*
Five or fewer minutes apart	Active labor *Time to head to the hospital or birth center, or call your midwife.*

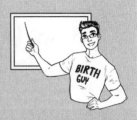

WHY STAY HOME DURING EARLY LABOR?

Many of the birth partners I work with express anxiety about hanging out at home after early labor has started. I've had more than one Dad say to me, "I'd feel better if we were at the hospital, just in case things start moving quickly." I hear what they're saying. If you've never had a baby before, it can feel a little frightening to experience a big chunk of labor without medical personnel nearby. Nevertheless, there are major advantages to steering clear of the hospital when Mom is working through the early stage of labor:

- *Mom can rest in her own bed.* If it's late in the evening and Mom goes into early labor, one of the best things she can do is sleep, if the contractions will allow it. The more rest she gets, the more energy she will have for the work ahead. You should rest as well. Mom is not going to be the only one awake and working hard.

- *Both of you can eat and drink.* Food will most likely be off-limits for Mom when she gets to the hospital. And food won't be readily available for you, Dad, so nourish your-selves while you can and get in a yummy meal or two.

- *Mobility is maximized.* After reading the last chapter, you are a mobility expert, right? I probably don't have to tell you that staying at home is going to help Mom remain as mobile as possible. She can walk around the block, go to the mall, or bounce on an exercise ball to her heart's content.

- *You can have more fun!* Think about all of the things you can't do in a hospital: have sex, host a dance party, play with your pets, go to your favorite restaurant, sing karaoke…you get the picture.

- *Friends can hang out.* Early labor is a fun time to gather together close friends or family and show Mom support while the contractions are still light enough to easily breathe through. Of course, if you and Mom are more introverted, you might want to hibernate and enjoy your last bit of quiet time as a couple.

- *Mom can take a bath or even go for a swim.* Not all hospital rooms have bathtubs, and water might feel really soothing to Mom during the early labor stage. This is a great time to have a good soak.

- *You won't be sent home for being an early bird.* If you go to the hospital before active labor has started, you are likely to be sent packing and told to come back once labor has progressed. If you want to save time and energy, hold off until labor has progressed to the more active stage and your doctor has given you the thumbs-up to drive to the hospital.

Using Soothing Words During Labor

Even when you choose to stay in the comfort of your home for early labor, Mom could probably still use some soothing. Let's talk about what you can do to be a supportive partner and to help Mom stay calm.

I explain to dads and birth partners that their number one objective during early labor should be to help Mom feel relaxed, happy, and distracted. We don't want her to start watching the clock or getting super anxious about what is ahead. We don't want her to start *benchmarking*—comparing her labor to that of others and feeling pressure to make things go a certain way.

If Mom starts saying things like "When is this baby coming? I've been doing this pregnancy thing for forty weeks! When in the world is this baby coming out?" it's time to pull out your Jedi-like skills. (Notice I wrote "skills," *not* "tricks." We're not tricking Mom. We're soothing her.) In the *Star Wars* movies, Luke Skywalker and the other Jedis use mind-control skills to influence people's behavior or to make objects float, right? That's not what we're doing here—we're not making Mom float. What we *are doing* is using mind-control skills to help Mom feel peaceful. Calming words, frequent distraction, and staying busy (the both of you) are the main tools you are going to use during early labor.

Let's face it, it's hard to see someone you love experiencing pain. You might find yourself feeling anxious and wondering how you can help. Mom might start acting testy or impatient. It is important to remind yourself and your partner that Mom's body is doing exactly what it needs to do: opening up the exit door and preparing for birth. Unlike other pain and suffering, this is good suffering. If you can remain calm, strong, and patient, you can really help to anchor Mom's mood and outlook.

MIND-CONTROL SKILLS—THE FIVE BE'S

Early labor is the time to let your Jedi-like spirit shine. I encourage birth partners to tap into these five "be's" when coaching Mom through early labor.

1. Be reassuring. It's normal for Mom to feel anxious and to begin doubting her abilities to get through the labor. What you can say: "This is exciting, honey. We're going to have a baby in the next day or so. I know you are feeling anxious, but your body is doing exactly what it is supposed to do."

2. Be loving and kind. This is the time to pull out some extra tenderness, especially if Mom usually responds positively to comforting words and compliments. What you can say: "I am so proud of you for carrying our baby. I love you and I'm going to stick by your side through this process."

3. Be patient. Mom might get testy. Mom might even snap or yell at you. Remind yourself that her body is literally opening up to deliver a human into the world. I don't know about you, but I might feel a tad grumpy if that was happening to my body! What you can say: "I know you're feeling frustrated and anxious. I know you are experiencing pain. Let it all out. I'm not going to take any of it personally. I am going to be here, no matter what."

4. Be strong and confident. Strength and confidence are the biggest gifts you can give to your partner during the labor and delivery. If she feels like you have her back, if she feels like you believe in her, she is going to feel calmer and more convinced that she can get through the birth. What you can say: "The doctor said that we should hold out until your contractions are a little closer together. You are doing great. I've got your back and will let you know exactly when it is time to head to the hospital."

5. Be distracting. Notice I didn't say "be distracted." Now is not the time to get lost in YouTube videos or the basketball game on TV. By "distracting," I mean initiate activities that will keep Mom's mind off the exact timing of her contractions and focused on how great she is doing. What you can say: "You know that house on the corner? Where they are doing all of the remodeling? Let's take a walk down there and see the progress they are making." Or, "Did we ever watch the last season of The Office? Let's watch it now. Dwight Schrute always makes you feel better, right honey?"

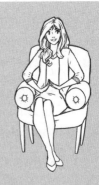

Counselor Corner: The Power of Your Words. Whether or not you are a *Star Wars* fan, there is plenty of evidence backing up Brian's claims that Jedi-like words can soothe and distract. In the 1970s, psychiatrist M. Erik Wright conducted a pioneering study regarding the power of healing words when used in medical emergencies. Dr. Wright divided a group of paramedics into two groups and asked one group to memorize a paragraph that included these phrases:

> We are taking you to the hospital. Everything is being made ready for you. Let your body concentrate on repairing itself and feeling secure... We're getting there as quickly and safely as possible. You are now in a safe position. The worst is over. (Acosta and Prager 2002, 8)

Half of the paramedics in the study recited the paragraph to their patients in the ambulance. The other half, the control group, talked to the patients as they normally did and didn't use any specific words. The results were pretty astounding. After six months of collecting data, Dr. Wright found that the patients who heard the script were more likely to survive the trip to the hospital, more likely to have shorter hospital stays, and more likely to experience quicker recovery rates.

The takeaway? Your words are powerful. They are soothing, reassuring, and maybe even healing. Mom's body will be more relaxed when she hears calming and confident words coming from her partner.

Staying Busy and Distracted During Early Labor

Britt and Sara chose to deliver their baby at a birth center with the help of a midwife. When Sara began having contractions, about twenty minutes apart, Britt checked in with the midwife.

"Sounds like Sara is just starting early labor. Why don't you two go get something to eat? Watch some TV. Take a nap. Give me a call again when those contractions remain consistently five minutes apart for about an hour. I'll be on standby. Exciting times!" the midwife told her.

"Roger that," Britt said. When she hung up the phone, she and Sara decided to go to the movie theater down the street and watch a comedy that had just come out that week. It was one of those fancy theaters that serves food, so they both ordered a full meal and fueled up for the adventure ahead. When Sara had a contraction during the movie, she squeezed Britt's hand and Britt recorded it on a tracking app on her phone.

When they got home, Sara started crying; she said she was feeling nervous. Britt hugged her and reassured her that they were completely prepared for the birth and that Sara would be amazing. Britt encouraged Sara to take a warm bath and to relax as much as possible. While Sara was soaking, Britt made sure their bag was ready to go to the birth center. Two hours later, they were on their way to meet their midwife, and six hours later, they were holding a gorgeous little boy.

Britt and Sara shared their birth story with me during a breastfeeding consultation. I loved hearing that they went out on a date during Sara's early labor and saw a movie that made them laugh so hard that Sara almost peed her maternity pants. From what Sara reported, Britt remained calm and confident, which allowed Sara to relax and ease into her labor. Britt kept Sara sufficiently occupied so that she didn't fixate on how many contractions she was having or the work that was ahead. Britt was in the zone, taking his Jedi-like skills to the max!

Many of the activities that Britt and Sara took part in during early labor are exactly the things I encourage my couples to do. Staying busy and having fun are key. Here are some early labor ideas that I usually give my clients:

Refer to a list of favorite activities. Remember that list of activity ideas that I encouraged you to make in chapter 2? This is a great time to pull it out and choose something fun to do. Maybe there is a great movie coming out that you want to see? A favorite restaurant that you want to treat yourself to? A mall or a store that you enjoy window-shopping in? Or a TV series that you want to binge-watch? As long as you're staying occupied and having fun, you are on the right track.

Have sex. Yup, I just said the "S" word. You might think this is a strange activity to embark upon during early labor, but if your partner is up for it and your doctor hasn't restricted sexual activity, intercourse is a great way to get labor moving along. Semen contains a hormonelike substance called prostaglandin, which may help to soften, or ripen, Mom's cervix. Having an orgasm may help spur your partner's uterus into action. Making love can trigger the release of oxytocin, a hormone that helps contractions progress. If nothing else, you're having fun and enjoying a little bit of intimacy before heading to the hospital. This is a win-win for all involved!

Try perineal massage. The area between the vagina and the anus is called the perineum. During birth, this area may tear a little bit. Many people believe that massaging the perineum with natural oils (olive, coconut, or primrose) can relax and stretch the skin. In addition, it can bring pleasure, relaxation, and even orgasm to Mom, which can help move labor along. Some couples do this form of massage throughout the pregnancy. Some try it during labor. Ask your doctor or midwife about the proper technique for perineal massage, or research it on your own.

The most important thing is to be gentle with Mom and make sure that she is comfortable with the activity. Relaxation and pleasure are key. With massage or any other soothing or sexual activity, I always encourage partners to use the "halfway rule." Use half the pressure that you would normally use, go half the distance that you would ordinarily go, and let Mom communicate whether she is comfortable with more.

Massaging the Perineum

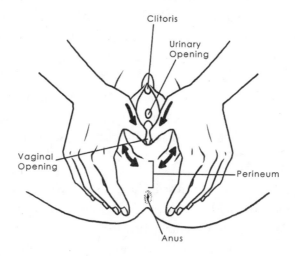

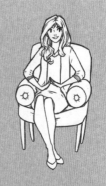

Counselor Corner: Taking Mom's Lead. Just as Brian said, it is important to follow Mom's lead when it comes to physical intimacy and interventions. Your partner might feel more vulnerable or sensitive during her pregnancy or labor. She might welcome physical intimacy and touch. Or she might push you away. Remember that the number one goal during labor is to help Mom feel safe and supported. Asking her what she is comfortable with and not pressuring her into any activity, regardless of how beneficial it might seem, are two actions that will help her feel like you have her back and that she is secure.

Eat and drink. As we discussed previously, early labor is a great time to get Mom as nourished as possible. After she arrives at the hospital, her food and beverage intake might be limited. So have plenty of her favorite drinks and snacks available and ready while you guys are at home. One idea is to buy her favorite protein bars ahead of time, chop them into small pieces, and put them in a glass jar or a ziplock bag. This makes it easy for Mom to snack on them. The extra protein will give her energy for the hard work ahead. Give Mom her favorite cold drink with a straw so she can take small sips on a regular basis. Smoothies or protein drinks are a great way to combine hydration and nourishment. If Mom is drinking lots of liquid, encourage her to visit the toilet frequently. Some birth professionals believe that a full bladder can get in the way of labor.

Breathe. We are going to discuss breathing exercises in more detail in the following chapter. However, early labor is also a great time to do some deep breathing. (In fact, any time during the pregnancy is a good time to do relaxation breathing.) I encourage clients to try five-five-five breathing when they are attempting to relax or calm down. Inhale to the count of five. Hold your breath to the count of five. Then exhale to the count of five. Do this five times in a row. I encourage both Mom and Dad to participate. When we humans are feeling anxious or excited, we often forget to breathe. This puts our body into fight-or-flight mode, which increases our anxiety. Taking in a full dose of oxygen and completely exhaling the carbon dioxide will make you feel like a true Zen master, I guarantee it.

Rest. I can't say it enough, but both of you should try to get some rest, be it at night or during the day. Although movement and activity can help the labor to progress, early labor is a good time to restore and reserve energy. If the contractions are light enough and Mom wants to lie down and sleep, encourage her to do so. When the contractions get stronger, she'll be up and ready to get to business!

Early labor can be a really special and exciting time for couples if they participate in some favorite activities and enjoy their time together. Use your Jedi-like skills to set the tone for the entire labor. Your partner and you will head to the hospital or birth center feeling confident and excited.

Reasons to Go to the Hospital Quickly

Now that I've encouraged you to chill out and relax during the early labor stage, I'm going to confuse you and tell you that there are a few instances when Mom might need to get to the hospital more quickly. Ha, ha! Just throwing you a little curveball. There are really only a few circumstances, so don't worry too much about them. I just want you to be informed.

Circumstance #1: Mom's water breaks. The technical term for this is rupture of membranes. What does it mean? The protective amniotic sac that surrounds the baby springs a leak. Although the movies would have you believe that there is a big torrential flood, usually the amniotic fluid leaks out of Mom's vagina as more of a slow trickle. Mom's water breaking before the birth occurs in only 15 percent of pregnancies and usually toward the end of labor (Gabbe et al. 2017).

If Mom's water breaks before labor has begun, it is important to contact your doctor or midwife immediately. Mom and the baby run the risk of developing a bacterial infection called chorioamnionitis if the baby remains in the sac too long. The doctor might instruct you to head to the hospital or to check the color of the liquid. If it's greenish or brownish, your doctor will probably have you head to the hospital more rapidly because the meconium (your newborn's first stool) is present in the amniotic fluid. If the liquid is clear or light yellow, your doctor might tell you to take your time getting to the hospital.

Circumstance #2: Mom has a preexisting condition or is diagnosed with a pregnancy complication. If Mom is dealing with a preexisting condition or a pregnancy complication, such as preeclampsia or gestational diabetes, you will probably be aware of it before labor begins. In fact, you probably will have already met with Mom's doctor or a fetal-maternal specialist to discuss how to proceed with the delivery. Your medical team will take great care to ensure that Mom and the baby remain safe. For this reason, they might ask Mom to arrive at the hospital before early labor begins. I will discuss preeclampsia and other pregnancy complications in great detail in chapter 7.

Circumstance #3: Mom experiences rapid labor. Rapid labor, also referred to as precipitous labor, generally only lasts between three to five hours. We've all heard stories about moms who gave birth in the taxicab on the way to the hospital or delivered their baby on the kitchen floor. Well, let me reassure you, as a doula who has attended hundreds of births, I can tell you that rapid labor is extremely unusual. It occurs in less than 3 percent of deliveries (Harms 2004), and it usually does not happen with Mom's first baby. That being said, if Mom's contractions come with no breaks in between, or if she yells that the baby is on the way, call 911. A responder can coach you through the birth process and send emergency personnel to help out. In chapter 7, I will prepare you for the highly unlikely possibility that you have to conduct an emergency delivery on your own.

Calm Early Labor Can Lead to Successful Active Labor

Okay, now that I have gotten your blood pumping a little, let's take some deep breaths and circle back to Lamar and Tonya, the exuberant couple I told you about at the beginning of this chapter. After I got off the phone with Lamar, I packed my doula bag and headed over to their house to hang out with them during early labor. By the time I walked in their front door, Lamar had completely changed his tone and was handling Tonya's early labor like a pro. There were candles lit in the family room and *Will & Grace* was playing on the TV. Tonya was sipping a protein smoothie and rocking in a glider. Lamar's voice, which had been loud and boisterous over the phone, was calm and almost a whisper as he filled me in on Tonya's contractions. "Ten to fifteen minutes apart but not very consistent," he explained. "I checked in with our doctor's office. The nurse told us to relax at home until Tonya's contractions are closer together."

I surveyed the scene and told Lamar that he was doing great. "I think you have things under control, sir. I'm going to duck out and hang tight until her contractions are five minutes apart and you send me a text," I explained, as I scooped up my bag and headed for the door. "Keep doing what you are doing, Lamar. Use those Jedi-like skills and soothing words. You're going to be a Dad soon. I'm super proud of you."

I meant it. I was really proud and impressed with Lamar's ability to calm down and take control of the mood while Tonya worked her way through early labor. He was definitely setting them up for success, and it showed when it came time for Tonya to deliver their baby. She was able to breathe through her contractions and give her full attention to pushing, both of which she credited to Lamar's calm and steady coaching throughout the day.

BG FINAL SHOTS

✔ *Unlike what we see on TV and in the movies, early labor can take a long time.* Follow your doctor's or midwife's directions and stay at home as long as you can. Use this special time to enjoy some favorite activities and pamper Mom before she heads in for the delivery.

✔ *Your words are everything.* What you say to Mom as she works through the various stages of labor can make a big difference. Channel some of your Jedi-like energy and use words that are soothing, reassuring, and confident.

✔ *When in doubt during early labor, communicate with your doctor or midwife.* Your doctor's office (or birth center) has people on call around the clock. Don't hesitate (or be embarrassed) to reach out to them if the labor seems to be speeding ahead or if Mom is experiencing any complications. Your birth team is ready and able to help and to answer any questions you might have.

CHAPTER 5

Supporting Your Partner Through Active Labor

When I was eleven years old, my youth pastor, Scott, taught me how to surf. I grew up near the ocean, and I was familiar with the ocean, but surfing the ocean was an entirely different adventure. When I examined the surf break with my pastor-turned-surf-guru for the first time, I found the rough seas scary as hell. The waves seemed to crash in random sets, some bigger than others, with no space in between.

Couples walking into the hospital to have a baby often feel as I did when I was first learning to surf. They might feel anxious about the unfamiliar setting and the birth itself. Mom's contractions might be coming in waves with increasing intensity. At times, Mom might feel like she is literally drowning in the pain.

When Scott and I paddled out the first time, wave after wave struck me in the face until I learned how to dive under them, like a duck, and breathe in between. Scott helped me to understand the mechanics of the ocean and how the waves had their own predictable rhythm. He taught me to not be intimidated by the force of the waves. The first time I caught a wave was exhilarating. Even though the waves were still powerful, and occasionally overwhelming, I felt a sense of calm control, like I could handle any intense experience in my life moving forward.

If you and Mom prepare for active labor, by familiarizing yourselves with the hospital (or birth center) and the mechanisms of labor, you too can feel this sense of calm control. If you learn and utilize a variety of tools to encourage breathing, distraction, and pain coping, you can help Mom to feel like she is diving under each contraction, breathing between them, and getting closer to that exhilarating experience of holding her baby.

Are you ready, Dad? Let's do this. Grab your surfboard, because we are about to plunge into the exciting sea of active labor. Before I give you all the tools you need to be a knowledgeable childbirth guru and a calming coach, let's talk about the journey that will lead you to the hospital and what to expect when you get there.

Time to Go to the Hospital

As we discussed in the last chapter, it's important to find out when your doctor or midwife wants you and Mom to report to the hospital or birth center for the delivery. In most cases, *if* Mom is having a healthy, normal pregnancy and her water hasn't broken, the hospital won't want to see you guys until Mom's contractions are five or fewer minutes apart.

There will probably be some other signs that Mom is ready to go. She might experience nausea and a loss of appetite. She probably won't be able to talk through her contractions. Mom should also expect to experience bloody show. Unlike losing her mucus plug, which is a gelatinous blob that usually falls out well in advance of the birth, *bloody show* is a gooey discharge tinged brown or pink by blood. Bloody show is definitely a sign that active labor is on the horizon.

Let's imagine the moment you decide it is time to head to the hospital: You've been hanging out at home and timing Mom's contractions. Your bags are most likely ready to go and by the door or in the car already. The distance between the contractions is hovering right around five minutes, and Mom is having a hard time talking though them. It's go time, right? Yes! But before you go anywhere, I want you to take a big breath.

From this point forward, it is of utmost importance that you stay calm and steady, Dad. Mom is going to feed off your mood and demeanor. If she feels your anxiety increasing, she might begin to feel panicky or out-of-control. You've been preparing for this day for months, so take a deep breath and remind yourself that you've got this.

TRAVELING TO THE BIRTH

The drive to the hospital or birth center is a great time to set the tone for the entire birth experience. You might have a five-minute trip or a thirty-minute trip. Regardless of how long your journey is, here are some suggestions for making the trip go more smoothly:

- *Opt for calming music instead of techno, heavy metal, or stressful news.* Try to create a spa-like atmosphere in the car. If Mom orders you to cut the music altogether, do as she says.

- *Have your route planned out ahead of time.* Use your favorite traffic app to double-check your path and make sure there are no traffic hazards or wrecks that will slow you down.

- *Don't speed or rush through stop signs and red lights.* There's no need to put the pedal to the metal, Dad. You'll most likely get there in plenty of time, and you don't need to get a traffic ticket on the way, right?

- *Think of any last people whom you need to call or text before the birth.* The neighbor who needs to let the dog out? The sister who is delivering donuts to the nurses? If Mom is able, she can make some of these last contacts while you are driving.

- *Keep the communication calm, positive, and flowing.* This might be the last private moment the two of you have before you are surrounded by beeping machines and helpful hospital personnel. Use this opportunity to tell Mom how excited you are to meet your baby, how proud you are of her, and how you know you guys are going to have an amazing experience.

Traveling to the hospital safely and serenely is going to set you and Mom up for a positive birth experience. Another important task is helping Mom to feel healthy and strong, *in spite of being in a hospital.* The story I am about to share with you illustrates how powerful and important this point is.

YOU'RE NOT SICK, MOM

Kate and Mason are two triathletes I partnered with in preparation for the birth of their first baby. These two were super fit. I was in awe of their muscle strength and endurance. They shared with me that they were planning for an unmedicated birth with very few interventions. Kate was confident and pumped, and Mason was ready to be a badass coach by her side. I had no doubts that they could make their plan a reality.

During one of our prebirth consultations, a tiny crack showed in Kate's otherwise rock-solid armor. She shared that she had been involved in a bad car accident when she was a teenager and spent more than two weeks in a hospital. She also talked about an amazing uncle whom she lost to cancer, and how his illness led to even more time spent at the hospital. For obvious reasons, Kate associated the smells and the colors— everything—of hospitals with trauma. Nevertheless, both she and Mason decided that they would feel more comfortable delivering their baby with nurses and doctors nearby. I validated Kate's discomfort. Then I arranged a long hospital tour so that Kate could familiarize herself with the space. She seemed to relax a little after getting a feel for where, and how, she would be giving birth to her baby.

When Kate went into active labor two months later, I met the couple at the same hospital. As I walked through the hospital entrance, a nurse was pushing out a wheelchair for Kate to sit in. I noticed an immediate change in Kate's demeanor after she sat in the chair. Her usually straight-as-a-board posture slumped slightly. Her eyes looked anxious, and her brow was furrowed. She clutched her bag close to her chest as she was wheeled down the corridor.

I knew we had to make a change. "Kate, how's your energy? Are you feeling good, feeling solid?" I asked as I walked alongside the wheelchair.

"Um...I'm okay, I guess. I don't know..." she quietly trailed off.

"How about if we get you out of that wheelchair and let you walk to the next room. You're strong. You've got this. Let's keep things mobile and talk about what is going to happen when we get to triage," I explained in an upbeat tone. "Mason, throw all of that gear you're hauling in the wheelchair. Let's use that thing as a luggage cart!"

The nurse laughed at us and the mood immediately lifted. Kate smiled and walked (okay, waddled) strongly down the hallway, pausing when she had a contraction. Mason and I winked at each other; we knew that we had the real Kate back and ready to rock the birth.

Some of the moms I work with love the wheelchair treatment—offer them a ride and they are ready to kick up their feet and roll. In Kate's case, I knew that it was important to not be treated like a sick patient. She needed to be reminded that she was at the hospital because she was about to deliver a healthy baby, not because she was fighting an illness or dealing with an emergency.

I see this scenario all the time with laboring moms. It is not unusual. As soon as Mom puts on her hospital gown or is attached to a fetal-monitoring device, her demeanor changes. The multiple wires and contraptions can make her feel weak and even sick. This is a key moment for you, Dad. Remind Mom that she is healthy and strong. She has been preparing herself and her body for this day for a long time. The monitoring is just part of the deal.

As I mentioned in the last chapter, the most powerful tools that you have in the birth experience are your words. Use them to reassure and encourage Mom from the get-go. Keep this in mind as you work your way through the different rooms and experiences at the hospital. In the next section, I'm going to give you a road map of what to expect at the hospital.

The Places You'll Go at the Hospital

When you enter the labor and delivery ward, you will definitely be stepping into "captain of the ship" mode. You'll be navigating the various rooms and advocating for Mom as you steer her through any choppy water. Mom will probably have a hard time talking through her contractions and might be focused on breathing in between them. For these reasons, she will need you to take the helm and assist with as much communication as possible. Here's a list of the various rooms you might visit and who you will encounter in each one.

CHECK-IN DESK

Just like you check in at a hotel, you need to check in at the hospital or birth center. If you preregistered, most of your info will be in the system. Have your credit card, insurance cards, and IDs read to show. If you are partnering with a doula, he or she might meet you at this spot. Be ready to do most of the talking, Dad. Mom will probably be working through her contractions.

TRIAGE ROOM

In smaller hospitals or birth centers, you will go directly to a labor and delivery room, but in a large hospital, your first stop will be triage, where patients are quickly assessed and next steps determined. The triage room is often a long, rectangular space with beds separated by curtains. Don't worry about the lack of privacy. This is just a temporary stopping place—you won't be getting super comfy here. In most cases, you and Mom will be transferred to your own private labor and delivery room after an initial assessment and intake.

Triage is where Mom will have a vaginal exam so a nurse can determine how dilated, or open, her cervix is. Her blood pressure, temperature, and other vitals will be checked as well, and she'll be attached to a fetal-monitoring device to check the baby's heartbeat and status. She might be connected to an IV or hep-lock. Remember, these types of interventions usually indicate that a person is very ill. As we just talked about, it is crucial for you to remind Mom that she is not sick and that these procedures are just part of the process. While all of this is happening, a labor and delivery room will be readied for the two of you—that is, if Mom is in active labor. If the staff determines that Mom is still in early labor, they might send you home to labor it out some more. However, if you and Mom waited until her contractions were five minutes apart, you are most likely staying put at the hospital.

There is one other thing that might happen in triage. The nurse might ask you to leave the room for a minute so that she can make sure that Mom feels safe and is not in an abusive situation. This is standard protocol for most hospitals. Don't feel offended or worried—you'll be back by Mom's side within seconds.

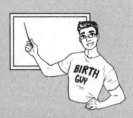
LABOR AND DELIVERY ROOM

The next stop on your adventure is the labor and delivery room, often referred to as the L&D room. You'll be spending the next few hours here, so go ahead and settle in. Set up your music. Take out your comfy blanket. Ready your tools, Dad. It's time to get busy! Of course, your number one priority is Mom. If she needs your attention or calming energy, toss your tools and bags aside and tune in to her. You're likely to have a pause between contractions to get out your supplies.

If Mom intended to have more mobility, she will probably get a hep-lock inserted in triage or in the L&D room. However, if she is being induced, is planning for an epidural, or has been diagnosed with group B strep, she will be set up with an IV.

I just mentioned something we haven't covered yet, right? Let me fill you in. Group B streptococcus (GBS) is a bacterial infection that may develop in a pregnant woman's vagina or rectum. This bacteria is found in 25 percent of all healthy adult women, so there's no cause for alarm (Edwards and Baker 2010). In other words, it's quite common, and a diagnosis doesn't mean that Mom is unhealthy or has a sexually transmitted disease. Occasionally, a Mom can pass the bacteria on to her baby during delivery, which can have severe consequences for the newborn. Therefore, Mom's doctor will test her for GBS between weeks thirty-five and thirty-seven of pregnancy. If Mom tests positive, the hospital staff will most likely administer antibiotics through an IV during the birth, which will drastically reduce the chances of your baby contracting GBS. If Mom was hoping for a hep-lock and not an IV, she might have to adjust the birth plan a little. The great thing about IV towers is that they have wheels, so Mom can still cruise around the room and make mobility a priority.

RECOVERY ROOM

In some hospitals, you will stay put in the L&D room throughout your hospital stay. It will become your little home away from home for a few days. But in larger hospitals, you and Mom might be moved into a recovery room after the birth. This will be set up with a bassinet for the baby, a bed for mom, and a comfy chair for Dad. If you're lucky, Dad, you might get a cot or a sofa bed to snooze on. This room is designed for exactly what it sounds like: recovering, resting, and getting to know your new baby.

OPERATING ROOM

You and Mom will only visit an operating room if she is scheduled for a cesarean section, or if the procedure is deemed necessary at some point during the labor. We'll talk all about C-sections in chapter 7.

Birth Guy Pointer: The Three Moods You Might Encounter at the Hospital. When you go to the hospital to deliver a baby, you are excited and exuberant, and you expect everyone you meet to be in the same state. Unfortunately, you won't always find that. Here are the three Cs that I frequently encounter in the hospital:

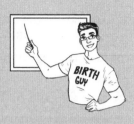

- *Cranky:* The clerk at the check-in desk might be working the eleventh hour of a twelve-hour shift. The triage nurse might have just been screamed at by a Mom in pain. Don't take it personally if the people you encounter are a little grumpy while communicating with you. Try a smile or a joke. Give them the benefit of the doubt and keep moving forward with your plan. They might just warm up a little after spending some time with you and your enthusiastic attitude.

- *Complacent:* Some hospital staff have been working in labor and delivery for years and are a tad jaded. Yes, you're experiencing the most important day of your life, but they really couldn't care less. Fortunately, these folks are few and far between. The good news is that people who are a tad complacent probably know what they are doing—they have a lot of experience. And again, they might perk up after spending time in your spectacular presence.

- *Compassionate:* I'm happy to report that *most of the time* you will encounter compassionate, nurturing, and enthusiastic nurses. These people have chosen labor and delivery services as their career, and the majority of the time, they love being there.

It's important to remember that the hospital staff and nurses are real people who might be dealing with their own stressors or issues at home. Try not to be reactive or to get angry if you have to deal with a grumpy or jaded person; some of the most effective nurses can be the ones who've seen it all before. Remember that it will only increase Mom's anxiety if she sees you in conflict or tense with the staff. If you really feel like your nurse is not a good fit, you can always dial 0 on the hospital room phone and ask to speak to the charge nurse. Let the front desk know that you are thrilled to be delivering at the hospital but that you don't think the nurse assigned to your room is a good fit. If the charge nurse is able, he or she will probably agree to assign someone else to your room. Most importantly, remember one of my earlier Birth Guy Pointers: having donuts, muffins, breakfast tacos, or cookies delivered to the staff always improves the mood across the entire ward. I've seen this in action. It works!

Working Through Active Labor

Okay, let's get back to what we are doing here at the hospital: helping Mom work through the most intense parts of her labor. It might be helpful to review what the labor is trying to accomplish with Mom's body. Remember that her cervix needs to open from zero to ten centimeters so your baby can safely exit the uterus. While the two of you were at home working through early labor, Mom's contractions probably helped her cervix open up to five or six centimeters. When you arrive at the hospital a nurse will check Mom's cervix and let you know exactly how open, or dilated, it is. Now that you are settled in your L&D room, her cervix needs to open up to eight centimeters during active labor. The last phase of labor, when Mom's cervix goes to ten centimeters, is called transition. Let me tell you, it is *quite* a transition. This will be the most intense part of the labor, and I will make sure you have plenty of tools to help Mom cope.

Because I know that all of the phases and stages of labor can begin to get jumbled in your head, below are some bullet points to help you keep it straight. If you and Mom are settled in an L&D room, you are probably done with the early labor stage. I included information about it anyway so you can visualize the entire labor journey. Visit http://www.newharbinger.com/41597 if you would like to print out a copy of this information in a chart format ("Stages of Labor Review: From Early Labor Through Transition") that you can have handy during labor.

Early Labor (Usually Experienced at Home)

- This stage lasts eight to twelve hours on average, but it can be much longer or shorter.

- There is usually five to thirty minutes of rest between contractions.

- The contractions (that is, the pain) generally last for 30-45 seconds.

- The cervix is dilated five to six centimeters.

Active Labor

- This stage lasts three to five hours, but the length of time can vary.

- There is usually three to five minutes of rest between contractions.

- The contractions (that is, the pain) generally last for 45-60 seconds.

- The cervix is dilated seven to eight centimeters.

Transition

- This stage lasts thirty minutes to two hours.

- There is usually thirty seconds to two minutes of rest between contractions.

- The contractions (that is, the pain) generally last for 60-90 seconds.

- The cervix is dilated to ten centimeters. (Time to have a baby, folks!)

What Do Contractions Feel Like?

Many dads ask me to describe what contractions feel like. I explain to them that just like the chocolates in Forrest Gump's box, contractions come in all shapes and sizes. Mom really doesn't know what she is going to get until she goes into labor. Moms have given me varying descriptions of what contractions felt like. Some say they felt like menstrual cramps on steroids, whereas others talk about extreme back pain. A lot of women describe an excruciating twisting and pulling inside their abdomen. Sometimes the pain was so extreme that they felt like vomiting. Most moms agree that the more they tensed up or fought the discomfort, the worse the pain felt. When they relaxed, their body and let the pain move through them instead of resisting, the contractions tended to work more effectively. I'm not going to lie—relaxing when you are feeling the most excruciating pain you've ever felt can be challenging. This is really hard work for Mom. I'm going to give you plenty of tools you can use to help her distract herself from the intensity and truly relax, but before we do that, let's talk about the ultimate pain-relief option: medication.

Pain-Relief Meds

We've talked about epidurals, but there are other pharmaceutical options that Mom might want to consider for pain relief. Or she might want to avoid medication altogether. As I mentioned already, we don't want to stand in a place of judgment about Mom's pain tolerance or preferences for pain relief. I encourage couples to explore options with their doctor prior to labor, so that they feel like they go into it fully informed. Here are a few of the options that a doctor might mention:

- *Systemic medications* affect Mom's entire system, not just one area of her body. They include painkillers, such as narcotics, and tranquilizers, which can help Mom to cope with anxiety or extreme nausea. Although they don't limit Mom's mobility entirely, they can cause her to feel sleepy, which typically leads to less movement.

- A *spinal block* accomplishes the same thing as an epidural, causing numbness in the lower half of Mom's body. It differs from an epidural because it is injected directly into the spinal fluid and is a onetime injection instead of a continuous feed through a catheter. It is faster acting than an epidural, but the pain relief only lasts a few hours, so it is frequently given when a Mom decides she wants pain relief late in labor. Sometimes, spinal blocks are combined with epidurals.

- *Epidurals* deliver continuous pain relief to the lower half of Mom's body. The medication is channeled through a catheter inserted into Mom's back. Approximately two-thirds of moms who have a hospital birth end up having an epidural. It's a safe and effective way to manage pain while allowing Mom to stay awake and alert. As we discussed before, the major downside is that Mom's mobility is limited after she has an epidural, which can cause the labor to last quite a bit longer.

WHEN TO REQUEST PAIN RELIEF

If Mom decided, prior to going into labor, that she wants an epidural or other pain-relief medication, note it on your birth plan and let the triage and L&D nurses know as soon as you check in. However, if Mom wants to labor it out for a while, encourage her to do so, and let the nurses know that you will alert them if Mom changes her mind and wants some relief.

I explain to all of my clients that there is no guarantee with any pain-relief options. Occasionally, an epidural will not take and Mom will still experience pain on one side of her body, or all over. Other times, the labor progresses so rapidly that there is not enough time to administer pain relief. It is a good idea to practice the various pain-coping strategies described in the next section, just in case Mom finds herself in one of these situations.

Coping with Pain

At least once a month I teach a Facilitating Fearless Birth class to a room full of couples. I explain to them that they should learn and practice multiple pain-coping techniques, because they don't *really know* what is going to help Mom until she is actually in labor. Additionally, one intervention might help with pain for a period of time, and then stop being effective a few contractions later. The best approach is to bring a bag full of tricks, figuratively and literally, and pull them out as needed.

I like to lead my clients in an exercise called the "ice holding activity." Have you ever held ice in your hand for longer than a few seconds? Take it from me, it's pretty uncomfortable. Of course, it is nothing like the pain of contractions, but it gives Mom a safe amount of pain and discomfort to experiment with.

Here's how it goes: I give both Mom and Dad a small handful of ice and challenge them to hold it for one minute. I ask them to report the level of discomfort they are experiencing. Next, I teach them different pain-coping strategies, which they then practice while holding the ice. This is a great way for Mom to see if any of the techniques resonate with her. Moms and dads both are able to hold ice longer and report less pain when they use some of these strategies. Pretty cool, huh?

Counselor Corner: A Scientifically Proven Pain-Coping Tool. Many of the pain-coping tools that Brian teaches revolve around distraction—turning Mom's brain away from the pain by having her focus her attention on something else. Neuroscientists have proven that distraction not only diverts the mind, it actually sends signals that block pain from reaching the central nervous system. In a 2012 research study, subjects were split into two groups and given memory tests (Buhle et al. 2012). The first group was given an easy 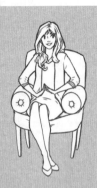 test, and the participants in the second group were given a more complex test that caused their brain to work harder. While they were taking these tests, they were subjected to a burning sensation on their arm. It was not hot enough to burn or mark their skin, but it did hurt. (Doesn't sound like a whole lot of fun, does it!) The researchers monitored their brains using functional magnetic resonance imaging (fMRI) while all of this was going on. The group that was given the more complex test reported less pain— the fMRIs showed that their brains were more preoccupied and their pain receptors were blocked. In fact, the researchers discovered that concentrating on something other than the pain caused the body to release opioid-based compounds that intercepted the pain receptors. This was an exciting discovery for the researchers, and it's useful knowledge to keep in mind when helping Mom practice pain-coping techniques. Some of these strategies might feel silly or weird, but they might just be the perfect tool for distracting and occupying Mom's attention when she is in the middle of a killer contraction.

PAIN-COPING TECHNIQUES

Here are some of the strategies that I teach couples in my class. I also utilize a lot of them when I'm in the L&D room with Mom and Dad.

Choose a focal point: Find an object that Mom finds visually soothing and enjoyable. It could be a photo of a family member or a favorite vacation spot. It could be a stuffed animal or some other sentimental item. Bring whatever Mom chooses to the hospital and encourage her to stare at it and to "get lost" in it during a contraction. You can also tell Mom to imagine herself zeroing in on the object and turning away from the pain. When the contraction ends, encourage her to come back from the object of her focus, back into her body.

Listening games: Ask Mom to listen to things close to her body, then to things far away from her body. Have her shut out the close sounds and listen for the far sounds. Then instruct her to shut out the far sounds and listen for the close ones. Yes, this sounds like something that stoned teenagers might have a lot of fun with, but I promise that it can be helpful for Mom as well.

Guided visualization: There is a multitude of apps and free websites that can lead Mom through a guided relaxation. Research them and try a few out at home so Mom can choose her favorites before going to the hospital. She might like the visualizations that take her through a rain forest or close to crashing waves. Or she might like a progressive muscle relaxation script that systematically directs her to tense and then release all of her muscles. If you've never tried one of these guided relaxations, Dad, I highly recommend that you give one a shot. Just describing them makes me feel more relaxed.

Personal touch: Massage, hugs, cuddling, and general touch can be incredibly soothing for some moms. If she enjoys plenty of touch when she is not in labor, there is a good chance that she will appreciate it during labor. Physical touch can lead to a decrease in the stress hormone cortisol and an increase in oxytocin, the hormone that impacts feelings of trust. Touch is powerful stuff, right? Massage, in particular, can distract Mom's brain and pain receptors from the contractions and put her focus on the pleasurable sensations of gentle pressure. Of course, it is always important to follow Mom's lead in regard to touch or any other intervention.

Rebozo techniques: Remember that long, colorful scarf that I told you to buy in chapter 3? Well, it's time to pull it out. There are countless ways to use a rebozo to ease Mom's pain. I've created a video ("Rebozo Techniques for Active Labor"), which you can view at http://www.newharbinger.com/41597, demonstrating multiple techniques.

Breathing exercises: Ask Mom to practice a visualization in sync with her breath. Encourage her to imagine herself pushing the pain away from her belly with her exhalation and breathing in relief with her inhalation. Mom can also try simply paying attention to her inhalations and exhalations, meditation style. If her focus wanders, encourage her to bring her attention back to her breath.

Dancing: This is one of my favorites. You and Mom went to the effort to make a favorite music playlist, so you might as well get up and groove to it. I encourage couples to slow dance with Mom's arms resting on Dad's shoulders. When she has a contraction, she can lean into you or press the crown of her head against your chest. Faster, playful dancing is great as well. The movement and rocking back and forth are going to help that baby cruise on down the canal.

Use all of your tools: Remember all of those things I directed you to pack up in chapter 3? Don't forget about them. This is the time to pull everything out and see what helps. Mom might want to drape herself over the exercise ball or do rebozo exercises on it. The warm water bottle might be a lifesaver when she is feeling the contractions deep in her back. Now is the time to put a few drops of lavender or peppermint oil on a cool towel and drape it around

Mom's neck. If you have a peanut ball, and Mom has had an epidural, your nurse can help you place the ball between Mom's legs so that it helps to open up her cervix.

Variety is so important when tackling active labor. As I said before, we don't really know what is going to help Mom until she is in the thick of it. Mixing up your approaches will help you to figure out what really helps Mom and also help her to move into different positions. The most important thing is to listen to Mom and to respond to her needs and wants.

Transition

Transitional labor, or *transition*, is the period of time when Mom's cervix dilates from eight to ten centimeters. This phase of labor is absolutely a metamorphosis, an evolution that brings you and Mom closer to meeting your newborn, and it can be beautiful and intense.

Transition typically goes quickly—in less than two hours. Mom's contractions will be longer, stronger, and sometimes completely overwhelming. For these reasons, you will probably see a shift in Mom's behavior and mood. She might hit a wall and insist that she can't do this "labor thing" anymore. She might thrash her body around and tear her hospital gown off or even rip up her sheets. Mom might seem frantic or angry. Occasionally I see moms get lost in what I call the zone, a place of extreme focus.

This can be scary for you, Dad. You might be wondering, *What the hell is going on! Where did my wife go?* It is important to remain calm and to remind yourself that those last two centimeters of opening are intense and transformational. Things are going exactly as they should be. Mom is just responding to the pain and the powerful transition she is experiencing.

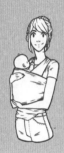

Mom Moment: Letting Go and Surrendering. Mom may get to the transition stage of labor and feel like she is literally dying, like she just can't deal with the pain anymore. The truth is that, in some ways, the person she used to be *is dying*. In that hospital room, in that exact space, she is literally transitioning from a woman to a mother. This is an empowering metaphor that many midwives and doulas share with moms and dads. There is no more powerful a transition than that to parenthood. Her life will forever be changed, and so will yours, Dad. If Mom can embrace the change and surrender to the process, literally letting go of her old self, she will move through transition more smoothly and quickly. Relaxing and allowing the contractions to do their work, instead of fighting them or trying to control the experience, is key. I know this sounds like heady stuff, but I encourage you to share this old birthing wisdom with your partner. Later on she might just say, "Wow, you were right about that surrendering stuff."

Regardless of Mom's behavior during transition, your role is to stick by her side and remind her that her work is almost done. She is on the last stretch; she is going to be holding her baby soon. Hearing that she is in transition and that her cervix is doing that last bit of work to get her ready for pushing can provide her the extra motivation she needs to hang in there.

MIX UP YOUR WORDS

When I think about transition, I think of Marci and Felix. I met up with them in triage and learned that Marci had already dilated to six centimeters. Her labor was going much more quickly than the couple had anticipated. By the time Marci was settled in the hospital room, she had progressed to seven centimeters, and although she had planned for an epidural, she decided to keep laboring it out. She was in the homestretch, right?

When Marci got settled in her room, she became really quiet and calm, to the point that it seemed like her labor had stopped altogether. This is something I've witnessed with a lot of moms. It's like Mom's body is giving her a quick breather before the most intense work of transition begins. Marci reclined on her side, closed her eyes, and rested. She looked angelic.

This little breather gave Felix and me a chance to catch our breath and prepare for the next stage, which we knew would be intense. We didn't have to wait long. Within a few minutes, Marci's contractions were back. She writhed in pain and moaned loudly, sometimes letting out an animal-like shriek. Felix was by her side saying, "You're okay, baby. You're doing great. You're okay, baby. You're doing great."

He must have said those two phrases twenty times before Marci screamed, "I'm not okay you S.O.B.!! STOP SAYING THAT!"

I let out a giggle when I heard this. I see this interaction a lot. Dad is trying *so hard* to be supportive, but he keeps saying the same phrase over and over. It almost turns into an annoying chant or mantra. When Marci was about to throw Felix out of the room, I pulled out the index cards that I use with dads and showed him different things to say in that moment.

I encourage you, Dad, to buy some index cards or sticky notes. Write down different encouraging phrases that you can say when Mom is in the thick of labor. Or create a list on your smartphone or tablet. Here are some of the phrases I have written on my index cards:

- I love you so much.

- I'm so proud of you.

- Your body is working through transition, which means it is almost time to push.

- You look really beautiful right now.

- You are so strong. Wow.

- I'm so excited to start our family.

- Pretty soon you'll be holding our baby. You are in the homestretch.

- You are rocking these contractions. You are working so hard.

- I know you are in a lot pain. That's a sign that your body is doing exactly what it should be doing.

- You are going to be an amazing mother.

- Let those contraction open things up. Remember to breathe. You're phenomenal.

- The nurse says that you are doing amazing. I'm really in awe of you.

- We are almost there. I am so excited. We're going to be holding our baby soon.

If you mix up your words and phrases, you are less likely to annoy Mom and more likely to encourage her. However, don't be surprised if she tells you to shut up altogether. As I've said before, the most important thing during active labor and transition is to follow Mom's lead and to keep your cool. We don't really know how things are going to be until we get in that L&D room. Going with the flow and keeping variety in the mix are part of what will make you a star labor coach, Dad. You and Mom will be moving into the pushing and birth phase before you know it. (If you'd like a more comprehensive list of things to say, visit http://www.newharbinger. com/41597 and download "Birth Guy's Sample Phrases to Say to Mom During Labor.")

BG FINAL SHOTS

✔ *Familiarize yourself with your hospital or birth center before the birth so that you know what to expect when you get there.* The more prepared that you and Mom are, the more confident you will feel when curveballs are thrown your way.

✔ *Variety and flexibility are key to helping Mom work through active labor.* We don't know what her experience is going to be until she's in the thick of it, so responding to her needs and trying different strategies will help both of you to stay afloat.

✔ *Transition can be intense and raw, but it is a sign that your baby is almost here.* Not unlike a beginner surfer, Mom might feel like she is being pummeled by waves and unable to breathe. If you remain strong, confident, and steady when Mom feels like she is about to lose it, you will help her to feel like she is riding the waves and getting closer to holding her beautiful baby.

CHAPTER 6

Pushing, Childbirth, and Beyond

There is a blue box that sits in the corner of most labor and delivery rooms. Much of the time, it goes unnoticed by the laboring Mom and her partner. I tend to keep my eye on this box. When Mom is nearing the end of transition and getting closer to full dilation, a scrub tech or nurse opens the box and begins preparing for the birth. It contains sterile supplies and childbirth tools. In my opinion, it holds much more than supplies—it contains optimism and encouragement. When we see that box opening up, we know that Mom is in the homestretch and about to deliver a baby. The unsealing of this box is monumental and exciting. Watch for its opening, Dad, because it will give you a much-needed boost of hopefulness as well.

As the grand opening of the blue box indicates, we've arrived at the most exciting part of the birth experience. I've witnessed an unbelievable number of births, and I have to tell you, they never lose their magic. Seeing a baby being born is one of the most amazing and life-changing events you will ever witness. In the following pages, I am going to give you a Birth Guy–certified, GoPro-style description of what to expect during this incredible chapter of your birth experience.

Mom Is Complete

If you hear a nurse say "Mom is complete," you might wonder, *What the heck is* complete? Mom is still writhing in pain and there is no baby in sight, right? "Complete" means that Mom's cervix is fully effaced (thinned out) and fully dilated (opened up) to ten centimeters. When these two things happen, Mom is through transition (Whew!) and ready to push. It's time to have a baby, guys!

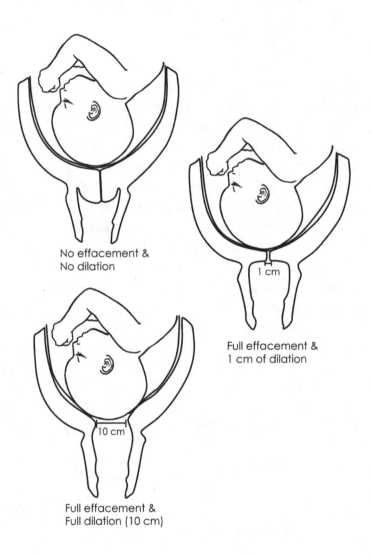

No effacement &
No dilation

Full effacement &
1 cm of dilation

Full effacement &
Full dilation (10 cm)

Who Is in the Delivery Room

When the blue box is opened and things are being prepared for the birth, new people will suddenly begin appearing in the room. These folks are supposed to be there—they all have a job and a purpose. Most of them will be wearing scrubs and surgical wear. Sometimes a doctor will put on galoshes. (Yup, childbirth can be kind of wet and messy.) Don't feel anxious about the presence of all these people. You and Mom just keep doing your thing. Here are some of the folks you might encounter during the birth:

- *A scrub tech or birth tech:* Similar to a nurse, these individuals are in charge of handling all of the equipment and assisting the doctor. They usually retrieve items out of the blue box.

- *A second nurse:* You've gotten to know your L&D nurse pretty well, and hopefully you've grown fond of her. Don't be surprised if another nurse (or two) is called in to assist with the delivery. The more helping hands, the better.

- *An anesthesiologist:* If Mom has an epidural, an anesthesiologist might be in the room during the birth to monitor the catheter or decrease the amount of medication she receives in order to help her push.

- *Your ob-gyn:* Believe it or not, this might be the first time you have seen your doctor since Mom went into labor. This often surprises my clients. They've gotten to know the doc so well over the past nine months that they're surprised she or he isn't a bigger part of the labor process.

In most cases, your doctor won't swoop in until Mom is ready to push and deliver a baby. Why? Well, he or she might be on call or tending to other births. To be honest, there isn't much for a doctor to do while Mom is working through her contractions. Most doctors usually wait for the final event and make a splashy (excuse the pun) entrance.

If it is a weekend or an overnight shift, you might get the doctor on call instead of your doctor. No need to worry—I've never met a doctor who didn't handle a birth with the utmost care and skill.

- *A perinatal team or pediatrician:* If there are any concerns about your baby's health that were discovered during the pregnancy, there might be a few extra doctors on hand to assess and tend to the baby as soon as he or she is delivered. Again, don't let their presence make you anxious. They are here to be helpful and to make sure your baby is as healthy as possible.

- *Your doula:* If you decided to partner with a doula, he or she has probably been with you throughout the labor and will most likely stay until your baby is latching on to Mom's breast.

Birth Guy Pointer: Who Else Do You Want in the Room? As I just described, when you give birth at a hospital, there are a whole heck of a lot of people in the room with you. If you hired a birth photographer to capture the birth, this person will also be occupying some space. Keep all this in mind when considering whether to invite family 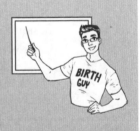 members or friends to attend the birth. It is going to be tight quarters in the delivery room! It is also important to consider the personalities and dynamics of individuals before inviting them. Childbirth is a beautiful experience, and you definitely want to share it in some way with loved ones. I just encourage you to think carefully before you offer any invitations. Make sure that any attendees will add to the experience and won't mind squeezing in with the rest of the crowd in the room.

It's Time to Push

Even though Mom's cervix is completely dilated, it is going to take major effort to get that baby out. Pushing can take anywhere from thirty minutes to an hour, but sometimes much longer. Mom will probably feel the urge to push on her own, unless she has had a spinal block or an epidural. For this reason, doctors will often have the anesthesiologist back off the epidural a little bit so that Mom can more easily push.

What does the urge to push feel like? To put it simply, most moms say that it feels like they need to poop...the biggest poop ever, with an enormous amount of rectal pressure. Not only will she be feeling pressure, but Mom's contractions will continue. This surprises some moms; they expect contractions and pushing to be two different experiences. Nope. The contractions continue and Mom will often be directed to push right along with the contractions. This can be excruciating but also extremely powerful. Mom might experience a burst of energy or a second wind at this point. She wants to get that baby out, right? She's ready to do this thing!

PUSHING POSITIONS AND HINTS

For many decades, the standard practice for pushing was to have Mom lie on her back in a hospital bed and push along with her contractions. This method is convenient for doctors because they get a clear view of the baby and easy access to the birth canal. However, this position is not always comfortable or easy for Mom. I still see many doctors directing patients to push in this manner, and it works—the baby definitely makes his or her way out. Nevertheless, I've been seeing a trend of doctors letting moms push and deliver in different positions. Many of these positions take advantage of gravity, which makes sense, right? Here are some of the more common positions:

- on hands and knees

- squatting with the help of squat bars

- sitting up

- lying on one side

- using a birth stool

More and more doctors are also letting their patients direct their own pushing. In other words, if Mom feels the urge to push, she pushes. This method allows Mom to follow her own instincts. During your prenatal visits, ask your doctor about his or her philosophy on pushing and what the hospital prefers.

Mom Moment: Pooping and Peeing During Pushing.
It's something that most moms fear and fret about the most in terms of pregnancy: Will a BM or urine make an appearance during pushing? Chances are, yes. Mom is being instructed to push as if she is having a bowel movement, so if there is anything left in her bowels, it will probably be coming out as well. Here's the deal: there will be a lot going on in the delivery room, and if 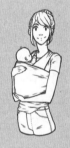 a little poop comes out, the doctor or a nurse will whisk it away or wipe it up—no harm done. Doctors and nurses have seen this a gazillion times, and they know what to do. In most cases, you and Mom won't even notice that it has happened. If Mom wants to avoid this happening in the delivery room, she should drink lots of liquids and try to empty her bowels prior to going into active labor. But there are no guarantees that poop won't make an appearance. Pee and farts can also emerge at any time. With all of that pressure, everything is being squeezed out. Again, neither of you are likely to notice because you will be so wrapped up in the intensity of the experience. Birth is truly raw, real, and beautiful. This is an opportunity for Mom to release all of her inhibitions and for Dad to show unconditional love and appreciation.

If Mom or the hospital prefers directed pushing, Mom will probably be told to push three times with each contraction, and then rest between contractions. Mom will be offered a mirror so she can watch what's happening when she pushes. This will help her to see her pushing in action. A nurse or doctor can also let her know if the pushing is working effectively. Mom might say, "NO way do I want to look in that mirror!" Or she might love the idea of seeing what's happening. As with everything else, leave it up to Mom to decide.

Some babies nearly self-eject—moms can hardly keep them in. It is not unusual for a nurse to tell Mom to slow down her pushing so that the baby's head doesn't come out too quickly. Other times, pushing takes *a lot* of time and energy. The baby might get stuck in a certain position for a little while. Shifting positions can help the baby to get unstuck and start going in the downward direction.

For directed pushing, the steps usually go something like this:

1. Wait until a contraction starts.

2. Take a deep breath and hold it; don't let it out.

3. Curl your chin to your chest and imagine yourself curling up around your baby.

4. Put your hands behind your legs and pull your legs up.

5. Push as if you are having a bowel movement.

6. Push for ten seconds and then exhale.

7. Repeat one or two more times during the contraction.

8. Rest until the next contraction. (This is key. Mom is working her butt off. Resting in between pushing will help her to build momentum for the next surge.)

WHAT IT LOOKS LIKE DOWN BELOW

When Mom starts pushing and the birth is about to happen, the doctor might turn on an overhead light, similar to a dentist's light, in order to get a better view of what's going on. I like to refer to this moment as "The Vagina Show," because the vagina truly is in the spotlight. Some dads like to go "south" and take a look at what's going on, but others prefer to stay "north" and focus on supporting Mom. Don't feel like you have to make a decision now about what you want to do. Follow your instincts when it's happening, and don't be surprised if a primal urge kicks in and you want to see your baby emerge.

I often warn dads that Mom's vagina will look extremely swollen and red. You might also see some blood and tearing. This can be a little scary, but I promise you that Mom's body has been designed to do this work. Right now it is focused on ejecting a baby, and it has a lot of work to do. My suggestion? If you decide to head south to take a peek, try to avoid saying things like "Holy shit! *What is that?*" or "Is it supposed to look like that?!" or "Oh… Wow…" For obvious reasons, statements like these will only increase Mom's anxiety. In this very moment she needs you to continue being supportive, positive, and nonreactive. We don't want her worrying about anything other than giving birth to your baby.

When you look below, you might also see the top of your baby's head, and even some hair. This is referred to as crowning, and it is an exciting moment. You can encourage Mom to reach down and gently touch the top of the baby's head. This touch can release a shot of oxytocin, which will give her extra energy to keep on pushing.

Just because you see the top of the baby's head doesn't mean that he or she is coming out immediately. It might take several more pushes. In fact, you might see the top of baby's head go in and out several times before the entire head comes out. Fortunately, Mom's body has been producing a hormone called relaxin that keeps the baby's bones and joints loose. Your baby's head will be able to handle the in-and-out action.

Counselor Corner: Sexual Trauma and Its Impact on Birth. Past sexual abuse or trauma can absolutely impact Mom's experience in the delivery room. She might feel exposed and vulnerable while pushing out a baby in a room full of people. She could feel out-of-control and even wonder about whom she can trust. It is not unusual for a Mom to have flashbacks due to the pain in her pelvic area and the positions she is being asked to get into. Occasionally, her labor will slow down or stall out due to the emotional shame or memories 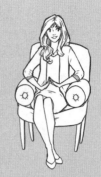 she is experiencing. These emotions can also affect a mom's ability to push her baby out. If a mom has a history of abuse or trauma, I encourage her to work with a counselor during the pregnancy in order to thoroughly process the trauma and prepare herself for the birth. There might be certain birthing positions or phrases that she would like to outlaw in the delivery room, and that is okay. I also encourage the couple to choose a birthing environment that feels safe and empowering. A doula can be extremely beneficial for these moms. A doula can act as an advocate, protector, and comforter-in-chief alongside Dad. In many cases, the birth can be a healing and empowering experience, an opportunity for a mom to take back her power and embrace her femininity and strength.

WHEN THE BABY WON'T BUDGE

Occasionally, a baby will stall out in the birth canal, and no matter how much Mom pushes, the baby will not emerge. Sometimes getting up and changing positions can help to shift the baby. When the baby is coming through the birth canal, we want the nose facing down, or toward Mom's back. If the baby is sunny-side up, facing Mom's belly button, the delivery might slow down. Some doctors will encourage Mom to lie on her side in order to help the baby flip over, like a pancake, to the right direction.

If Mom is absolutely exhausted, or if the baby needs to be delivered in a hurry due to fetal distress, the doctor might opt to use one or more tools to help the baby emerge. This brings me back to the blue box we talked about at the beginning of this chapter. The doctor might pull out forceps, which look like large salad tongs, or a vacuum extractor, which has a little suction cup on the end. If you see either tool being used, don't be alarmed. Both apparatuses are standard instruments that doctors have used for many decades to gently ease the baby's head through the birth canal.

In rare instances, regardless of the tools used, the doctor will not be able to coax the baby through the birth canal. Mom might have an extremely narrow canal, or the baby might be stuck in a strange position. If the doctor is concerned that the baby's safety, or Mom's safety, is in danger, he or she might whisk Mom off for a C-section. Again, this rarely happens. Mom's body truly is designed to do this work.

WHEN THE BABY IS BREECH

Most babies will move into the head-down, ready-to-go delivery position a few weeks prior to birth. When this fails to happen, the baby's bottom or feet, or both, might be positioned to be delivered first. This is referred to as breech presentation. Your doctor or midwife will usually discover that the baby is breech a few weeks before the birth. She or he can usually feel exactly where the baby's head and bum are by performing a simple exam of Mom's belly. If the baby is breech, Mom might choose to try a few natural things to turn her baby.

Maddie and David, whom I worked with, discovered that their little boy was breech when Maddie went in for her thirty-six-week checkup. Maddie immediately went home and began researching ways to turn her baby. She met with an acupuncturist a few times. She tried swimming and lying on her side. Nevertheless, that little baby wasn't budging. Although I am seeing a return to vaginal breech births, most doctors will encourage parents to opt for a

C-section if their baby remains feet down. Maddie and David decided to take their doctor's advice and go the C-section route. The birth of their son was still beautiful and amazing, even though it wasn't the plan they had envisioned.

If your doctor or midwife informs you that your baby is in the breech position, discuss your options. Although Maddie and David's little boy stayed feet down, many moms do have luck naturally turning their baby before the due date arrives.

The Birth

Okay, let's get back to that moment you've been waiting for. Your baby is about to come out into the world, and it really will be the most memorable experience of your life.

You've already seen your baby crowning. Your doctor might have dripped olive oil or baby shampoo over Mom's vagina to help the baby easily slide out. In spite of these lubricants, it's not unusual to hear Mom say, "It's burning! Burning!" This "burning ring of fire" sensation is caused by the skin and muscles stretching and even tearing a little around the vagina as the baby emerges. Although definitely uncomfortable, this experience is perfectly normal. Reassure Mom that she is just feeling the baby coming out and that the burning will go away as soon as the baby is delivered.

Usually there is one final push that sends the baby's head out, and then the body quickly follows. Mom will feel a slippery gush of a feeling and absolute, amazing relief. Don't be surprised if there are gasps, cheers, and tears all around.

There's some other stuff that emerges with baby—mainly a whole lot of liquid and bloody-looking stuff. Hence the galoshes that the doc is wearing. The baby has been living in a sac of liquid for months, and all of that liquid needs to emerge.

When the baby comes out, the doctor will quickly check to make sure the umbilical cord is not around the baby's neck. He might suction the baby's airway to clear it. If there are any concerns about the baby's health, the doctor will take immediate action, but in most cases, the baby will be handed to Mom for immediate skin-to-skin contact.

This is an incredible moment, guys.

Breathe it in.

Take a mental snapshot.

You are now officially parents, and I'm so effing excited for you!

CUTTING THE CORD

The umbilical cord, that long ropelike thing that connects the baby to the placenta, needs to be cut soon after the birth. As I mentioned earlier, many doctors and midwives are opting for delayed cord cutting so that the baby can continue to get nutrients for a short while after the birth. Usually, they wait for one to three minutes after the birth before bringing out the scissors. Then they will ask you to do the honors, Dad.

Don't be intimidated by this prospect. It really is quite simple. The doctor will hand you a pair of sterile scissors and show you exactly where to snip the whitish cord. Then he or she will put a small clamp on the end of the cord closest to your baby's belly. If you're hoping the doctor will make your baby a pretty belly button, I'm sorry to report that the doctor doesn't have much control over how it turns out. The appearance of a belly button, whether it is an "innie" or an "outie," has everything to do with how your baby's skin naturally heals on its own after the little umbilical-cord stump falls off.

If you have opted for cord-blood or placental-cell banking, the process of collecting stem cells for future medical use, you will have already informed your providers. Your doctor, midwife, or nurse will know how to properly capture and store the blood in collaboration with the storage service you are using.

THE BIRTH ISN'T DONE, GUYS

Mom still has a little bit of work to do. She has to deliver the placenta, but it will be much easier than delivering the baby. This is often referred to as the third stage of birth, and it is just as important as all of the other stages. The placenta can emerge anywhere from five to twenty minutes after the baby. This organ provided nourishment and comfort to your baby for the last ten months, but now its work is done and it has to be evicted. While Mom is holding the baby and getting amazing skin-to-skin contact, she most likely will be experiencing mild contractions that will help the placenta to break free of the uterine wall. I usually encourage Mom to sniff the top of the baby's head, which will give her a boost of oxytocin that helps loosen the placenta and starts her milk flowing. Occasionally, a doctor will give Mom a bit of Pitocin (a medication that is usually used to induce labor) to help get the placenta out. She might also tug gently on the umbilical cord to ease the placenta along. Mom will feel the placenta come out, but it will be a lot less painful than pushing out the baby. She might not even notice it exiting her body.

When the placenta comes out, the doctor will examine it to make sure all looks well. Remember that the placenta is actually an organ that Mom's body produced to take care of the baby. Amazing, huh? Let's all give some gratitude for the placenta. If all looks good, the doctor will wrap up the placenta and it will be discarded along with other medical waste. However, if you arranged ahead of the time to bank stem cells, encapsulate the placenta, or even make smoothies out of it, the doctor will put it in the container you brought for this purpose.

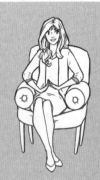

Counselor Corner: Postpartum Depression and Placentas.
Don't be weirded out by the placenta smoothie idea. Moms consuming their placentas in some form is actually a centuries-old practice. Some believe the placenta contains beneficial nutrients and minerals that can help Mom far beyond the pregnancy and birth. Many claim that consuming the placenta increases Mom's oxytocin, restores her iron levels, and supports her milk production, as well as stabilizes her mood.

Although there is some controversy about whether these benefits truly are a thing, I've heard many moms swear that consuming their placenta helped them ward off postpartum depression and fatigue. Does Mom cook up the placenta and eat it with a fork and knife? No! The placenta is carefully encapsulated by a team of professionals in your area. They usually steam, dehydrate, and grind the placenta into a powder that is inserted into capsules. Mom can ingest the capsules directly or add the powder to smoothies. Chat with Mom and your doctor or midwife about this option. If Mom is concerned about postpartum depression, placenta encapsulation might be a service that she wants to invest in. However, Brian and I both caution you to research the encapsulation service thoroughly. You want to make sure that the placenta is prepared and encapsulated in a sterile and professional environment.

STITCHING MOM UP

Following the delivery of the placenta, the doctor will examine Mom's vagina and birth canal for any tearing or birth trauma that occurred during the delivery. Mom just delivered a small human through her vagina, so there is a good chance that a little bit of tearing happened.

Doctors used to frequently perform episiotomies during childbirth because they believed that it allowed the baby a little extra room to emerge and prevented tearing. An *episiotomy* is a small surgical incision made to the perineum, the muscular area between the vagina and the anus, just before delivery, to enlarge Mom's vaginal opening. Doctors rarely perform episiotomies anymore because years of data have shown that allowing Mom's vagina to stretch naturally (and sometimes tear naturally) will do less damage and allow for better healing in the long run. Your doctor might still opt to do a small episiotomy if forceps or vacuum suction are deemed necessary. If this is the case, don't worry, Dad. Mom will heal completely with proper care and time.

Tears (or lacerations) in the perineum typically range from first degree to fourth degree. *First-degree tears* are the most common and involve the skin of the perineum and the tissue around the opening of the vagina, but no muscle. These tears are fairly superficial and only require a couple stitches, if any.

Second-degree tears go deeper, into the muscles underneath the perineum and vagina. These tears need to be stitched closed, layer by layer. They'll cause Mom some discomfort and usually take several weeks to heal.

Third- and fourth-degree tears are more severe and definitely require a substantial number of stitches and medical care. These affect less than 2 percent of women (Eskandar and Shet 2009) and can cause complications, such as severe pain and anal incontinence, for weeks after the birth. However, I don't want you to worry about this happening, Dad. These types of severe tears are very unusual, and if—on the off chance—they do occur, Mom's doctor will properly treat them and provide follow-up care.

Is there anything you can do to prevent tearing? Sure. You might not be able to prevent it entirely, but there are definitely things you can do to prepare Mom's perineum. Perineal massage, discussed in chapter 4, is a great way to help Mom's skin and muscles loosen up and possibly become more elastic before the birth. (And it feels good too!) Using lubricants such as olive oil or baby shampoo during the birth, and encouraging Mom to slow down her pushing, can help the baby to slide out more gradually and easily. In my experience, I have noticed that moms who have epidurals are more likely to tear, possibly because they can't feel the strength with which they are pushing.

Regardless of the degree of tearing, Mom will be given instructions on how to care for her perineum in order to maximize healing and minimize pain following the birth. The majority of moms are able to return to normal activity, including sexual activity, within six weeks after the birth.

AFTEREFFECTS OF BIRTH

Directly after the birth, the room will start to empty out. The doctor will finish up his tasks and bid you adieu. Only a nurse or two will remain, who will be tending to Mom and taking care of a few tasks with your baby. This is a good time to ask any family members or friends who attended the birth to go share the great news with those waiting outside. A break from visitors will allow the three of you some time to get acquainted and to work on breastfeeding.

This time will also provide you an opportunity to love on Mom a little. She just went through an enormous ordeal and is probably exhausted. The nursing staff will most likely bring her some food and drink to begin getting her nourished. A nurse or doula will be working with her and the baby to get breastfeeding off to a good start. For the next two hours, a nurse will come and massage Mom's abdomen every fifteen minutes. The goal is to help her uterus shrink and prevent Mom from developing blood clots. Here are a few other things that Mom might also experience following the birth:

- *Shakiness:* It is normal for a mom who just gave birth to shake and quiver like a bowl of Jell-O in an earthquake. This is a natural response to the immediate hormonal shifts that occur after delivery and a possible endorphin release. If Mom needs to walk across the room or take a shower, give her plenty of support and encourage her to use the shower bench so that she can easily maintain her balance.

- *Help in the bathroom:* The first time Mom uses the toilet, a nurse will probably help her steady herself and show her how to flush and soothe her lady parts using a "perineum bottle" filled with warm water. Toilet paper will feel like coarse sandpaper to Mom at this point, so the perineum bottle will be a lifesaver for the next few days. Most moms are given a stool softener to help them pass their first bowel movement after birth. That first BM can be a little scary for Mom. She just delivered a baby and doesn't want to experience any more pain or pushing down there!

- *Bleeding:* Mom is going to be releasing quite a bit of blood over the next few days and even weeks. Although this is a normal function of her body recovering from the birth, it can be overwhelming. The hospital will provide Mom with enormous pads and mesh underwear to catch the blood. They aren't the sexiest undergarments in the world, but they keep Mom comfortable and dry.

- *Contractions:* Believe it or not, Mom might still be experiencing mild contractions as her cervix and uterus shrink. If Mom received Pitocin, the contractions could be quite strong. Fortunately, they won't be as strong as the birth contractions and should dissipate fairly quickly.

- *Adrenalin high:* Regardless of how little sleep the both of you have had, you might find yourselves experiencing a jolt of adrenaline. Leave the Red Bull at home, Dad. You're going to be full of vim and vigor. There is nothing more exciting than welcoming your first baby into the world. You will probably be riding high for quite a while.

Let the Visiting Begin

After you and Mom have taken some time to enjoy your baby and work on breastfeeding (which I will go over in great detail in chapter 8), you might be ready to welcome all of those visitors back into the room. Feel free to ask them to enter in small groups. If it's late at night, you can even ask them to come back the next day. Ask Mom what she is up for, and follow her lead. The most important visitor will already be sitting by Mom's side: YOU.

You will have been Mom's birth coach and team player. Her cheerleader and her biggest fan. Give yourself a big ol' pat on the back, Dad. You are going to do an amazing job, I just know it.

BG FINAL SHOTS

✔ *Giving birth to a baby is raw, real, and incredibly rewarding.* There will be screams and grunts. There will be plenty of blood and bodily fluids. In the end, there will be a baby. It truly is a beautiful thing.

✔ *The show is not over after the baby emerges.* Childbirth is a multi-stage process. Mom will still need to deliver a placenta and possibly be stitched up. Continue to provide support and encouragement while Mom works through these final stages.

✔ *Mom will experience plenty of aftereffects following her delivery.* She will be counting on you to be her right-hand man as her body recovers and adapts to parenthood. Your bond will be stronger than ever after going through this incredible experience.

CHAPTER 7

Navigating C-Sections and Other Unusual Birth Circumstances

April had just reached the forty-week, full-term mark when she began having contractions. Usually, I would have encouraged her and Jared, her husband, to hang out at home and labor it out for a while, but April was experiencing concerning symptoms: significant swelling of her legs and severe stomach cramps. Both her doctor and I encouraged her to head to the hospital and get checked out. After noting April's high blood pressure, hospital staff gave her a room and began treating her for preeclampsia. They administered magnesium sulfate to get the preeclampsia under control and Pitocin to get her labor moving along and her cervix dilating. April and Jared had hoped and planned for a vaginal birth, so we all settled in and began working on getting that labor moving along.

Twenty hours later, April had only dilated to four centimeters. The baby hadn't dropped, and Mom was pretty exhausted. In addition, the magnesium sulfate was giving her extreme nausea and blurry vision. It was time to take a different course. April's doctor decided to prepare April for a cesarean section. Fortunately, Jared, April, and I had discussed and planned for this possibility. As Jared and I changed into the scrubs required in the operating room, I reminded the couple that they were in good hands and were still going to have a beautiful and meaningful birth experience. I gave Jared a high-five and told him that he was about to become a Dad. I reminded him that April needed him to continue being the top-notch birth partner that he had been during the last twenty hours. His work as chief supporter and encourager was definitely not complete. I reminded him that, most importantly, both April and the baby were going to be safe.

Most couples who hire me as a doula are pregnant with their first baby. They've never embarked on the childbirth adventure before and want as much guidance as possible. April and Jared were one of these couples. When I work with couples like April and Jared in the months leading up to a birth, I prepare them for the moments when things don't go exactly as planned. As with most adventures in life, it is great to visualize and plan for best-case scenarios. But, as we discussed earlier in the book, you also want to prepare for those times when things go off course. In this chapter, I'm going to fill you in on what I like to call the off-roading adventures of birth: C-sections, pregnancy complications, labor induction, premature births, and precipitous (that is, *really fast*) labor.

If you are heading down the pregnancy highway and encounter one of these obstacles, I want you to feel prepared to smoothly navigate the alternate routes you might have to take. By the time you finish this chapter, you will feel confident enough to support Mom through any unexpected detours during the birth experience. Let's begin with the most common off-road adventure, the cesarean section.

C-Sections

A *cesarean section* is the use of surgery to remove one or more babies from a mother's uterus. How does the surgery unfold? The doctor makes a six-inch incision in Mom's lower abdomen. Next, he makes a second incision in the uterus and removes the baby, placenta, and umbilical cord. Mom's uterus and abdomen are promptly stitched up and the healing and bonding officially begin. Approximately one out of three babies are born by cesarean section in the United States. That's a whole bunch of babies, so I want to make sure that you feel fully prepared if you and Mom end up in the operating room.

The cesarean is not a new medical procedure. There are accounts from some of the earliest civilizations—Egyptian, Chinese, and Roman—of babies being born this way. If you're wondering where the practice got its name, it is not entirely clear. Some say the word originates from the Latin *caedo*, which means "to cut." The doctor is technically cutting into a section of Mom, right? Others posit that Julius Caesar, or one of his sons, was born this way. To be honest, it doesn't matter where the term comes from. What matters is that the cesarean can be a life-saving procedure for both Mom and baby. Most people refer to the procedure as a C-section, but I affectionately refer to it as "vaginal bypass surgery." Mom is still giving birth, but the baby is leaving the body via an alternate path. Let me assure you, no badge of honor accompanies a vaginal birth. A new mother is a gloriously strong creature, and a baby is a beautiful blessing, regardless of which route he or she takes to enter this world.

WHY MOM MIGHT HAVE A C-SECTION

C-sections are usually deemed necessary when vaginal birth poses risks to Mom or the baby. There are many circumstances in which this could be the case:

- The baby is presenting breech (feet are pointing down toward the cervix) or is in another position that makes moving through the birth canal difficult.

- Mom is experiencing a *really, really long* labor and doesn't seem to be progressing.

- The baby is showing signs of fetal distress, such as a decelerating heart rate.

- Placental issues have been discovered, usually through ultrasound, such as placenta previa (the placenta is covering Mom's cervix and blocking the exit) or placental abruption (the placenta has separated from the wall of the uterus too early).

- The baby is really big. (Usually doctors will allow Mom to labor it out for a while, but if an especially large baby is not moving down the canal, a C-section might be necessary.)

- There are pregnancy complications for Mom, such as high blood pressure, preeclampsia, or other medical issues.

- The parents elected to have a C-section. There are various reasons why couples decide to go this route. Perhaps Mom already had a C-section or a traumatic birth. Maybe Mom is pregnant with twins or triplets.

Regardless of why or how a couple decides to have a C-section, I never stand in a place of judgment. How to give birth is a deeply personal choice that couples should decide with the help of their birth provider. I'll say it again and again: childbirth is beautiful and empowering regardless of how your baby enters this world.

WHAT HAPPENS DURING A C-SECTION

Let me pull out that GoPro camera again and show you exactly what you will encounter during a C-section. Even if you feel absolutely sure that your baby is going to be exiting through your partner's vagina, I encourage you to read this section, just in case.

The first thing the nurse will do is transfer Mom to an operating room (OR) and prep her for surgery. Before Mom is wheeled out, or if you get to walk with her, be sure to offer words of encouragement: "We've got this, Mama. You are going to be okay and I'm going to be with you. We're going to be holding our baby soon. I'm going to put on some scrubs and will be right by your side."

Once Mom is settled in the OR, an anesthesiologist will assess Mom's pain-relief needs. If Mom already has epidural anesthesia flowing into her, the anesthesiologist might use the same method to continue numbing Mom from the waist down. Or the doctor might administer a spinal block. Either way, the anesthesiologist is going to make sure that Mom doesn't feel an ounce of pain during the surgery.

While Mom is being prepared for the C-section, you, the birth partner, will be handed scrubs, a mask, a hat, and special booties. Don't forget to take your phone or camera into the OR. And definitely don't forget to take a quick selfie of yourself in your surgical gear—you're going to look totally MD in this moment.

Mom might be alarmed by all of the surgical clothing and gear. She might be emotional and tearful. Reassure her that the gear keeps the room sterile and protects her and the baby. Keep reminding her that she is in good hands and that she is going to be okay. Take big breaths if you need to, Dad. Remember, one out of three babies are born this way; it's going to be okay.

When Mom is settled on the surgical table, a drape will be placed between her head and abdomen, extending up toward the ceiling from beneath her breasts. This keeps the surgical area sterile and prevents Mom from seeing the surgical tools and the incision. In some hospitals, Mom's arms will be strapped down in a horizontal, or Christlike, position so she isn't tempted to try and grab her baby and touch the surgical area in the process. However, this practice is being phased out in most hospitals.

After the anesthesiologist has given the thumbs-up, the doctor will begin the procedure. The anesthesiologist will remain in the room, making sure that Mom stays comfortable. The doctor will make two incisions, one in the abdomen and one in the uterus, and you will see Mom's body jiggling a little as the doc reaches in and

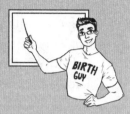
grabs the baby. The doctor needs to move rather quickly, so the process is not as soft and gentle as you might hope for. After the baby is out, the doctor will most likely show your new little one to Mom. This is a really magical moment. Some of the most amazing photos happen during C-sections, so be sure to snap a few pics. You guys are officially parents!

There is still plenty to do in that operating room. The doctor might allow you to cut the umbilical cord, Dad. She will also need to cauterize (or burn) Mom's blood vessels and stitch her up. You might smell a faint burning odor from the cauterization. Remind yourself that this is a normal part of the procedure.

This is important: If at any point you feel dizzy or faint, Dad, let a nurse or the anesthesiologist know. One or the other can grab a stool for you to sit on. Be sure to take deep breaths. The procedure will be over quickly. Focus on that cute baby. Focus on being there for Mom. You're doing great, Dad.

BIRTH PARTNERING DURING A C-SECTION

You might think that there isn't much for a birth partner to do during a cesarean section. This couldn't be further from the truth. During a C-section, your role as birth coach and partner is more important than ever. Here are some tasks that you can be doing for Mom.

Narrating for her. Mom can't see what's going on, and she definitely can't get up and move. You can help her by putting on your sports-commentator hat and sharing the play-by-play of what is happening during the birth:

- Looks like the doctor is preparing her equipment.

- Another nurse just entered the room. She's smiling. She's ready to do this thing.

- Okay, babe, they are going to get started.

- Oh, I think we are about to see a baby!

- Look at that healthy little guy coming out. Oh, he's kicking. Can you hear him?

- Oh, man, he is good-looking.

- Okay, they are taking the baby over to be weighed and assessed. I'm going to walk over there with them. I'll snap a photo for you. I'll be right back.

- Now they are stitching you up. Almost done, honey. You are amazing.

You get the idea, Dad. Keep up a running commentary so Mom is in the loop. This will decrease her anxiety and allow her to feel more involved in this amazing experience.

Advocating for her. Again, Mom will be lying flat and might feel overwhelmed by everything going on around her. If something feels odd to you, or if you have a specific request, be sure to speak up, Dad. You can be Mom's eyes, ears, and voice. Here are some examples:

- Do you mind turning down the music a little?

- Oh, wow, sounds like you all have great weekend plans, but could you share with us a little about how the procedure is going?

- Glad you had an amazing lunch, but my wife hasn't eaten in a while and I'm getting a little squeamish hearing about food. Mind if we change the subject to the baby?

- Is there any way that Mom can get some skin-to-skin contact with that cutie? I know she would really love that.

Capturing moments for her. Digital cameras and smartphones have changed everything in the C-section operating room. Now you can snap photos of what is going on and immediately share them with Mom. I don't necessarily mean photos of Mom's open flesh, but I do mean a photo of the baby emerging, a photo of the baby being weighed, and a photo of the baby on Mom's chest for the first time. As soon as you take these pics, show them to Mom so she can see what you are seeing. Sometimes your doula, a family member, or a professional photographer will be allowed in the OR. If this is the case, this person can handle the digital capturing and you can focus on Mom and the baby. Showing Mom photos in real time will help her to avoid feeling left out.

Walking for her. Mom won't be able to walk during the surgery, or for a while afterward. You are going to be adding up some major steps on your Fitbit, Dad. You'll be traveling over to the scale to watch your baby being weighed and swaddled. You'll probably carry your baby back over to Mom or back to the recovery room. You will be Mom's right-hand man, grabbing her water, blankets, or anything she might ask for. Wear some comfy shoes, Dad. You're going to be logging some miles.

Birth Guy Pointer: A Different Kind of Strength. As I mentioned in the last chapter, childbirth can be a primal experience that demands a certain kind of strength from Mom. In the delivery room, Mom pushes with all her might and might even feel a natural urge to pull the baby to her chest. A C-section requires a unique kind of strength 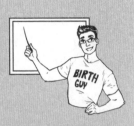 because Mom has to relinquish control and allow other people to deliver her baby. To give up this control, to go against these primal urges, takes a lot of strength and courage. Be sure to tell Mom how strong and brave you think she is. She's surrendering all control in order to safely deliver a child into the world. A person doesn't get much stronger than that.

After the baby has been born and checked out, the staff will allow you and Mom to have some time with the baby while they finish up Mom's stitches. They might hand you or Mom the baby in an odd position. When you lay the baby next to Mom, make sure your baby's head is aligned with Mom's head. It is important that she can see the baby and be as close as possible. Better yet, place the baby against Mom's cheek so that she can smell, kiss, and feel the baby. This will be calming for Mom. She will see that her baby is okay, and that she is going to be okay. The physical contact will get the oxytocin flowing, which will help Mom and the baby to bond and to get breastfeeding off to a good start in the hours to come.

RECOVERING FROM A C-SECTION

Even though Mom was fully awake during the C-section, she just had major surgery and will need plenty of time to recover.

Instead of the two days that new parents typically stay in the hospital, you and Mom will be staying three to four days. Try to enjoy these extra days at the hospital, Dad. The nurses will take good care of Mom and allow her to rest and bond with the baby. This extended stay will give her extra days to work on breastfeeding and allow her body to heal. This can be a time of rest for you as well. After you return home, Mom will need up to six weeks to fully heal from the surgery. Knowing this, it will be important to help her with any household tasks and heavy lifting. Enlist help from friends, family, and neighbors, if you need to. Be sure to add in rest and self-care for yourself so you can continue to be strong for both Mom and the baby. If the dishes or laundry begin to pile up, don't stress. You guys can get to them later. The important thing is to allow Mom to heal and rest while the two of you get to know your baby.

Pregnancy Complications

As you saw with the story of April and Jared, there are times when things may go off course with pregnancy, and Mom might need to be closely monitored, to have her labor induced, or to be scheduled for a C-section. I am going to give you a brief overview of some of the complications that I see in my practice. I share these not to worry you, but to give you enough info so you feel fully prepared to face them, if necessary. As I will explain, these conditions only occur in a small percentage of pregnancies. The key thing I emphasize to all of my couples is to *contact Mom's provider if she is having any concerning symptoms.* You won't be bothering your doctor or nurse, I promise.

PREECLAMPSIA

Preeclampsia, the condition that sent April to the hospital early in her labor, is a medical disorder characterized by high blood

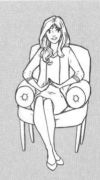

Counselor Corner: Coping with Grief When Things Don't Go as Planned. There are all kinds of postpartum grief that I see in my counseling practice. One of the more frequent forms of sadness I encounter is when a new Mom expresses grief that her birth didn't turn out the way that she had hoped. Perhaps she ended up getting an epidural when she planned to go without medication. Often, Mom will experience grief if she has an unplanned C-section. Mom might see this as some sort of failure on her part. Or, as Brian said, she might feel like she didn't succeed in earning the Vaginal Birth Badge.

These emotions are completely normal and to be expected. It is incredibly difficult when we go into an experience with expectations for a certain outcome, and things go awry. In sessions, I usually validate and normalize the grief moms (and sometimes dads) feel. Of course they feel disappointed and sad that things didn't go as planned. I also celebrate their strengths: these parents navigated unforeseen events and did the absolute best that they could in the moment. If your partner feels sadness or regret over the way things went down in the delivery room, don't immediately try to talk her out of her grief. If you allow Mom to process her very normal feelings, you can slowly ease into sharing all of the things that you believe were awe-inspiring and beautiful about the birth.

pressure, swelling of the hands and feet, and protein in the urine. It affects 5 to 8 percent of pregnancies and usually occurs during the second half of the pregnancy (WHO 2011). Doctors and midwives watch closely for this condition because it can cause serious complications, and even fatality, if left untreated. Every time that Mom goes in for a checkup, her blood pressure and urine will be checked. She will also be asked about headaches and swelling. Some swelling during pregnancy is normal, but a significant amount can be problematic. If your doctor detects preeclampsia, he might put Mom on bed rest or induce labor early.

Another preeclampsia treatment is an intravenous magnesium-sulfate infusion at the hospital. If your doctor chooses this treatment, he will probably warn Mom of some common side effects: headaches, blurred vision, and impaired balance.

Treatment for preeclampsia has come a long way in the last century. Your provider will watch for it closely and know how to handle it in order to keep Mom and the baby safe.

LOW AMNIOTIC FLUID (OLIGOHYDRAMNIOS)

Oligohydramnios is a long and intimidating word, but the meaning is quite simple: there is not enough fluid in the amniotic sac to protect and cushion the baby. This condition occurs in only 4 percent of births and usually shows up during the third trimester (March of Dimes 2013). The provider may suspect this diagnosis if Mom leaks small amounts of amniotic fluid, measures small for her stage of pregnancy, or does not feel the baby move very much. Other conditions, such as preeclampsia or diabetes, can also lead to low amniotic fluid. If a provider is concerned about Mom's fluid levels, she will most likely order an ultrasound in order to visually measure the fluid. If the diagnosis is confirmed, and Mom is far enough into the pregnancy, the doctor might induce her or schedule her for a C-section.

GESTATIONAL DIABETES

Between weeks twenty-four and twenty-eight, Mom will usually have a glucose screening at her provider's office. She'll be instructed to chug a sugary beverage in five minutes or less. Sounds like a fun game at a college keg party, right? Truthfully, most moms are not a big fan of this test. The drink contains fifty grams of glucose. It is syrupy sweet and makes some moms want to gag. One hour after finishing the drink her blood will be drawn to see how efficiently her body processed the sugar. If her blood sugar reading is too high, she will have to come back to the office on another day

Mom Moment: A Word About Bed Rest. Occasionally, a provider will diagnose a pregnancy complication, premature labor, or an issue with a mom's cervix and put her on bed rest. This can mean different things for different pregnancies. Sometimes bed rest is simply periodic resting, but other times, Mom will be told she literally *cannot leave the bed*, unless she needs to use the restroom or bathe. Bed rest can feel *extremely* challenging for an expectant mom who is eager to wrap up projects at the office, deep clean the house, or run errands before her baby arrives. Of course, the number one priority is keeping Mom and the baby safe. You can calm and reassure Mom by reminding her that everything else can 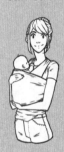 wait—her safety and health are of utmost importance. You can also help Mom by picking up the slack wherever you can. This will mean taking on household tasks and enlisting help from friends, family, and neighbors. Buy Mom a ton of fun magazines. Set up the TV and food tray next to her. Encourage her to relax and enjoy some pampering. Bed rest might feel like an eternity to Mom...but her baby will be here before she knows it, as will her return to activity.

and take a three-hour glucose-tolerance test to see if she has a temporary condition called gestational diabetes. Less than 10 percent of expectant mothers are diagnosed with this condition (DeSisto, Kim, and Sharma 2014). If Mom is one of them, she will work with her provider, and possibly a nutritionist, to develop an eating plan that will help her to manage the condition. The good news is that blood sugar returns to its prepregnancy state for most moms soon after they give birth.

PLACENTA PREVIA

Placenta previa is a condition in which the placenta lies low in Mom's uterus, next to or covering her cervix. In most cases, the placenta will mosey on upward later in the pregnancy, but occasionally, it refuses to budge. This can cause complications, such as bleeding. It can also cause the baby's exit, through the cervix, to be blocked. If placenta previa is detected during a midpregnancy ultrasound, Mom will be scheduled for a follow-up ultrasound. If the placenta doesn't shift upward, Mom might be scheduled for a C-section to safely deliver the baby. I rarely see placenta previa with my clients—it is present in only about one out of two hundred births (Ananth, Smulian, and Vintzileos 2003).

The complications that I listed above are the more common ones, and yet they occur in very few pregnancies. As I said before, I don't share any of the information to worry you but rather to inform you. The most important thing you can encourage Mom to do is to *go to her regular checkups with her health care providers*. They will run the tests, they will order the ultrasounds, and they will monitor Mom's health. You get to focus on being a strong and supportive partner. In most cases, a doctor's goal will be to keep the baby in Mom's womb for as long as possible, but if Mom has a complication that poses a threat to her or the baby, the doctor might decide to induce labor, which leads me to my next topic.

Inducing Labor

It's super warm and cozy in Mom's womb. If I were a baby, I definitely wouldn't want to leave. Nevertheless, doctors decide quite frequently that they need to give the baby a little nudge and get Mom's labor going before contractions have naturally started. This is called labor induction, and it happens in approximately one out of five births (ACOG 2009). There are various reasons why a doctor might decide to induce labor:

- *Mom is a week or two past her due date.* Although there is some debate about how long it is safe for Mom to go beyond her due date, most doctors will make the decision to induce if the pregnancy is nearing forty-one or forty-two weeks in order to ensure the safety of both Mom and the baby.

- *Mom's water has broken and her labor has not started on its own.* As we discussed earlier, if Mom's membranes have ruptured, there is a slight risk that she might develop an infection. In order to prevent this infection and keep the baby safe, most doctors will want to get the labor going if it hasn't started already.

- *Mom is experiencing a pregnancy complication (such as the issues we discussed earlier) or a health complication.* If the doctor feels like there is any serious risk to Mom or the baby, she will induce or schedule a C-section, sometimes long before Mom's due date if there is a serious enough risk.

- *Logistics dictate that the baby needs to get moving.* The parents might live a long distance from the hospital, and it might be too difficult for them to travel the distance when Mom naturally goes into labor. Or the doctor might be going on a Caribbean cruise in two days. If Mom wants her own doctor to deliver her baby, and Mom has reached or surpassed her due date, she might be induced.

HOW LABOR INDUCTION WORKS

First, Mom's health care provider or a nurse will determine the condition of her cervix when she arrives at the hospital. The provider will check to what extent the cervix has softened, effaced (thinned out), and dilated (opened up). Remember, Mom's cervix needs to thin out and open up to ten centimeters before she can deliver her baby. What the provider or nurse discovers during a pelvic exam will help determine which mechanical or medicinal methods will be used to "ripen" the cervix and get labor started. Here are some of the more common methods used:

- *Administering synthetic prostaglandins:* Prostaglandins are the natural hormones that help Mom's cervix to thin out and dilate. The provider might insert a gel with synthetic prostaglandins into Mom's vagina, or give the medication to her orally, to prepare the cervix for labor. Just this simple procedure can often kick-start contractions and get labor moving along.

- *Stripping or sweeping the membranes:* This is a fancy way to say that the provider inserts her finger into Mom's vagina and manually separates the amniotic sac from the lower part of her uterus. This will often cause prostaglandins to naturally begin flowing, and contractions may follow. Doctors frequently use this method in their regular office and then send Mom home to see if labor will start spontaneously.

- *Rupturing the membranes:* If Mom's cervix is already thinning out and opening, the doctor might insert a small hooked instrument into the vagina in order to manually rip open the amniotic sac and break Mom's water. This will often send a signal to Mom's body that it is go time, and contractions will begin spontaneously.

- *Using a synthetic form of oxytocin:* Oxytocin is the feel-good hormone that gets labor going. It is also the hormone that is released when someone is hugged, massaged, or has an orgasm. Oxytocin is good stuff! The synthetic form of oxytocin is called Pitocin, and it is the most frequently used method of inducing labor. Pitocin is administered through an IV. The presence of the hormone coursing through Mom's body will usually get labor going. Sometimes the nurse or doctor will increase the amount of Pitocin flowing through the IV if Mom's body is not responding.

Relaxing and allowing her body to surrender to the process can be the final things that help Mom's labor to be induced. Use your words and actions, Dad, to calm and reassure Mom. Give her a shoulder rub or a foot rub to get that natural oxytocin flowing. Tell her that you are amazed by her strength and courage. The induction will go more smoothly if Mom is feeling at ease and ready to embrace her labor.

If Mom has been induced due to a pregnancy complication or a health concern, chances are that it is early in Mom's pregnancy. I want you to feel fully prepared for the possibility of having a sweet little preemie, which leads me to the next topic.

Premature Birth and the NICU

Premature birth is defined as birth before thirty-seven weeks. Approximately one out of ten babies is born premature in the United States, which equals about 380,000 babies each year (Martin, Hamilton, and Osterman 2017). These babies are referred to as preemies and are often the most amazing little miracles.

Babies are born early for a variety of reasons. A doctor might decide to induce labor early because of health risks for Mom or the baby due to pregnancy or health complications. Other times, Mom might spontaneously go into early labor for unknown reasons. Regardless of the how or why, doctors and hospitals are ready and prepared to give preemie babies the best chance possible at surviving and thriving. Thanks to the work of researchers, dedicated doctors, and organizations such as the March of Dimes, standard practices and care for preemie babies have advanced at rocket speed in the last century. The vast majority of preemie babies go on to have healthy, normal childhoods and lives.

I will always remember my client Sofia and the precious preemie boy that she brought into the world. Sofia, an expectant single mother, hired me to be her doula for the birth of her first baby. I felt super honored to be given this opportunity, because I would act as her doula *and* her birth partner. Later, it was clear that the universe connected me with Sofia for a reason, because she encountered multiple challenges in both her pregnancy and birth story.

After a fairly uneventful first two trimesters, Sofia developed high blood pressure in week twenty-nine. Her doctor treated her for preeclampsia with medication and bed rest, both in the hospital and at home. Sofia also received a shot of steroids to strengthen her unborn baby's lungs, just in case she needed to be induced early. Sofia had her blood pressure regularly checked and her blood drawn. Unfortunately, her symptoms did not subside, and both her health and the health of her baby were at risk. When she was thirty-four weeks along in the pregnancy, Sofia's doctor decided to induce. I met her at the hospital, and we got ready to do some labor. Sofia was understandably scared and upset. I gave her big hugs and reassured her that she was in really good hands. I told her that I wasn't leaving her side.

After she got settled into her L&D room, Sofia's doctor manually broke her water and started her on Pitocin through an IV. When the little baby was born, he weighed in at just over three pounds. The doctor allowed Sofia and her little boy to have a short amount of skin-to-skin contact, and then he was whisked off to the NICU (neonatal intensive care unit) to be cared for and monitored. Sofia's baby spent nine days in the NICU. Today that little boy is a strapping toddler—you would never know he had been a tiny three-pounder at birth! The care that Sofia's little guy received in the NICU was phenomenal. Although Sofia admits that her time on bed rest and the birth of her baby were scary, she is so thankful for the support and care she and her baby received at the hospital.

THE NICU

The neonatal intensive care unit, more commonly referred to as the NICU, is a place of great care and love in the hospital. It is where the littlest and sickest babies go to heal and grow. Sometimes these babies finish out their second and third trimesters in a NICU incubator. Even full-term babies can end up in the NICU if they have serious health issues and need to be closely monitored or cared for.

It may feel scary and intimidating if your baby ends up in the NICU. Here are some of the things that I encourage moms and dads to consider.

The machines, technology, and people are there to help your baby thrive. A NICU is very different from a typical nursery in a hospital. There are incubators (enclosed, climate-controlled bassinets) and lots of nurses and doctors circulating. Feel free to ask as many questions as you want regarding what is going on with your baby and what the various machines are doing. In spite of the multiple contraptions and providers, the space is often soothing and calming.

It is common for preemie babies in the NICU to be dealing with serious health issues. Many preemie babies do not have fully developed organs, so their little bodies might struggle to adapt to the outside world. Breathing difficulties are the most common, as their lungs are trying to figure out how to take in air. Preemie babies can also develop heart murmurs or necrotizing enterocolitis, a condition in which intestinal tissue is injured or failing. Remember, the large amount of technology and the medical procedures in the NICU are designed to address these conditions and get your baby healthy. In most cases, preemie babies will heal and outgrow their issues as they get bigger and stronger.

Skin-to-skin contact and bonding are just as important as ever. Depending on how big your baby is, you might be able to touch him with your hand or hold him on your chest. Talk and sing to your baby so he can hear your voice. Express to the staff your desire to get as much skin-to-skin contact as possible. If you mimic a kangaroo, and keep your baby close to your warm skin, you will help your little one to heal and thrive.

Breast milk is still the best nutrition. If your baby is big enough to digest milk, the NICU staff will help Mom to express milk and feed your baby through a small tube—even if Mom's breast milk seems like it's nowhere near coming in.

Birth Guy Pointer: All About Milk Banks. Many people are not aware of the nonprofit banks all over the country that store and distribute breast milk. Generous mothers who have a surplus of pumped milk donate it to the banks, where it is pasteurized and sterilized in order to make it completely safe for preemies and newborns. These banks distribute the milk to families with preemie babies or to moms who, for a variety of reasons, are unable to get their milk supply going. If your baby comes early, and Mom is not able to express any milk, ask the hospital staff, perhaps a hospital social worker, about your local breast-milk bank. The tiniest bit of colostrum (extremely nutritious milk that comes the first few days after birth) or breast milk can give a preemie baby a much better chance at surviving and thriving.

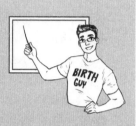

YOU are part of your baby's care team. If your baby ends up spending time in the NICU, it will feel like a bizarre new world at first. But very quickly you will learn the rhythms and the responsibilities of everyone and everything in the unit. Keep in mind that you play a big role in making decisions and planning for your little one's care. Ask to be involved when the docs and nurses discuss the clinical care plan for your baby. Speak up and ask questions when something seems odd or when you see inconsistencies with your baby's care. Most importantly, take care of yourself and encourage Mom to do the same. It is crucial that you rest and keep your energy up so that you feel strong and prepared when it's time for your baby to come home. If either of you are struggling with grief, depression, or anxiety, ask to speak to a social worker, chaplain, or counselor. Care for yourself, please, so that you can care for that sweet, tiny baby!

Your end goal: Bringing your baby home. The minute your baby enters the NICU, this question will probably be foremost on your mind: When can we take our baby home? In order for your little one to head out the door, she needs to be able to function in the outside world like a full-term baby. She needs to breathe on her own, maintain her body temperature, and swallow and digest milk. The hospital wants to get your baby to this place as much as you do. Try to relax and take advantage of the extra care and comfort in the NICU while your baby is building her strength and her organs are developing fully. Your baby will be heading home as soon as the staff can allow her to do so.

Precipitous Labor

There is one last unusual birth circumstance that I want to touch on before closing this chapter. It is the type that we frequently see in the movies and hear about on social media but rarely see in real life: the *really fast* birth. *Precipitous labor* leads to birth less than three hours from the start of contractions. It makes up less than 3 percent of deliveries (Harms 2004). Moms are more likely to have a fast birth if they have a superefficient uterus, an extremely "compliant" birth canal, an especially small baby, or a history of rapid birth.

How does a Mom know that she is having precipitous labor? The contractions might abruptly start coming with no breaks in between. Mom might feel the sudden urge to push and be unable to stop. She might scream out, "Baby's coming!" Or she might just scream. Or she might calmly announce that the baby is on the way. No matter what, you'll be able to tell that she is serious and that the baby is coming.

Counselor Corner: A Word About Fetal Demise. The loss of a baby is a delicate subject to discuss with expectant parents. Both Brian and I usually only say a few words on this topic when we meet with pregnant couples. We don't want to worry clients, but we do want them to know their options and feel prepared if they face a fetal loss, *or* if they know other parents who have experienced the death of a baby. When a baby passes away in utero during the first half of a pregnancy (before twenty weeks), the loss is referred to as 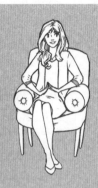 a miscarriage. When parents lose a baby during the second half of a pregnancy (after twenty weeks) or during labor or birth, the loss is referred to as fetal loss, fetal demise, or stillbirth. Both categories of loss can be devastating and very hard to prepare for. In the United States, there is a less than 1 percent chance that a couple will have a stillborn baby (Cousens et al. 2011). Parents often discover this loss when their baby stops moving or kicking in the womb. An ultrasound will confirm whether their baby has a heartbeat.

If the baby dies while still in the womb, the sad truth is that Mom will still have to go through the birth. Her body may spontaneously go into labor, or she may be induced. Regardless of how the unborn baby is delivered, the hospital staff has been trained to explain your options and care for Mom, Dad, and the baby with sensitivity and tenderness. Now I Lay Me Down to Sleep is a lovely nonprofit that provides professional photography services in the hospital to parents who want to capture images of their sweet baby. The hospital will typically provide a memory box in which you can keep a lock of hair and a footprint. As a counselor, I don't make assumptions about how these couples will grieve or how they will want to remember their baby. I meet them where they are at and join them on their journey of grief and recovery. I usually find that talking about their baby and their loss is an important part of their healing. If you, or someone you know, experiences a miscarriage or a stillbirth, please reach out for information or support from a counselor or supportive organization in your area. There are many of us who are ready and willing to talk, listen, and simply be with you.

Although it is highly unlikely that you'll have precipitous labor, I want you to be prepared if you do. Think like a Boy Scout, right? Here are the steps you can take if Mom announces that the baby is coming and you don't have time to get to the hospital or birth center:

1. If you are in a car, pull over to a safe place and call 911.

2. If you are not in a car, have Mom lie down or recline (so the baby doesn't fall out) and call 911. Make sure the front door to your house is unlocked. If you have time to wash your hands, do so.

3. Try to remain calm and encourage Mom to breathe, or even pant like a dog, to slow down her pushing. Pushing the baby too quickly might cause Mom to tear, so encourage her to take her time. It's probably a good idea for you to take some deep breaths as well, Dad.

4. Continue to calm and reassure Mom: "I'm right here. You're going to be okay. Help is on the way. You're amazing. I'm not going anywhere. We can handle this, honey."

5. When the baby starts crowning, and the head emerges, gently cradle the side or back of the baby's head. Do not pull on the baby's head or neck or put a lot of pressure on the top of the baby's head. Mom's body will eject the baby. Your job is to carefully catch your little one. Mom's primal instincts might show up in the moment, and she might reach down and grab the baby herself.

6. If the umbilical cord is around the baby's neck, gently slip the cord over the baby's head without tugging on it.

7. When the baby emerges, he or she should start breathing and will usually let out a cry. Rub your baby's back to gently stimulate breathing, if necessary.

8. Place the baby on Mom's chest and wait for the paramedics to get there. Do not pull on the umbilical cord or placenta.

9. Take a big breath! You're a Dad! And you are amazing.

Okay, that was a bit of a roller-coaster ride, wasn't it? Chances are that you won't need *any* of the info that I gave you in this chapter, so let's just call this the "Just in Case" chapter. Now that you've read it, tuck all of the information away and know that you can pull it out if and when you need to.

BG FINAL SHOTS

✔ *A C-section can be just as beautiful and intense as a vaginal birth.* How you coach Mom through the procedure and how you embody the advocate role will make all of the difference in the quality of the experience.

✔ *When in doubt during the pregnancy, call your doctor or midwife.* If Mom is feeling weird or if something doesn't seem right, make the call. Your provider can determine if an issue needs to be addressed or if Mom needs to go to the hospital. You get to focus on taking care of Mom and yourself.

✔ *The vast majority of pregnancies and births go off without a hitch, but you want to be prepared for potential off-roading adventures*—just in case. Kudos to you for completing this chapter. Hopefully you won't encounter any of these circumstances, but if you do, you will be prepared to act, unlike many birth partners out there.

CHAPTER 8

Your New Baby and Breastfeeding Basics

We spent the last seven chapters preparing you to deliver a baby into the world. You've learned about morning sickness, early labor, and C-sections. Now…we finally get to talk about your newborn baby! In this chapter, I'm going to share with you what to expect immediately after your baby is born. I'm also going to give you the complete insider's scoop on breastfeeding.

Believe it or not, many couples skip this step in their parenting preparations. They take the childbirth classes, they set up a beautiful nursery, but they gloss over learning how to care for and feed their baby after he or she has entered the world. Yes, you and Mom will learn *a lot* as you go, but I'm not going to let you go into the experience without a beginner's guide. Before we dive into the fascinating subject of breastfeeding, I want to go back to the hospital room and prepare you for what will happen immediately after the birth. Are you ready? Here we go!

Meet Your New Baby

Let's turn our attention to the wonderful being who is lying on Mom's chest directly after the birth. Although the number one priority will be skin-to-skin contact and you and Mom having the opportunity to admire the new life you just created, there will be a few other things that will be happening. The cool thing is that your birth team knows how to complete these tasks in a nondisruptive and gentle manner so you'll barely know they are happening.

THE APGAR SCORE

Your baby won't be going to school for several years, but he'll be getting his first grade in the hospital. Virginia Apgar, an obstetric anesthesiologist, developed the Apgar test in 1952, and it has become the standard tool for assessing newborns in a hospital setting. The Apgar provides a quick overall assessment of the baby's well-being, providing measures of the baby's color, heart rate, reflexes, muscle tone, and respiratory effort. A score between 0 and 10 is given immediately after the birth and at the one-minute mark, and it determines if the baby needs immediate medical care. A score between 7 and 10 means that the baby only needs routine care. A score between 4 and 6 means that the baby might need some assistance with breathing. A score under 4 usually indicates that the baby needs prompt life-saving measures and will most likely be transferred to the NICU.

The test is repeated again at the five-minute mark, and again every five minutes if the baby's score falls below 7. Let me reassure you, just because your baby gets a low Apgar score at birth does not mean that he will be in poor health later.

In my many years as a doula, I've rarely seen Apgar scores below 7. I also *never* see a 10. The doctors refuse to give A+ scores, guys, so don't fret if your little one doesn't get a perfect 10. Your baby can still be perfect in your eyes.

WHAT IS THAT WHITE STUFF ON MY BABY?

When your baby emerges from the birth canal, she might look a little odd. She'll probably be covered in a white waxy coating called vernix. In the twentieth century, it became common practice to bathe newborns immediately after the birth. Now most providers simply rub babies with a soft towel, leaving most of the vernix on the skin. Why? Well, vernix is kind of amazing. It protects the baby from germs, it helps to maintain body temperature, it moisturizes the skin, and it contains that wonderful new baby smell that helps Mom and the baby to bond. Let the white stuff stay, Dad. It might look funny, but it really is benefiting your baby.

BABY'S ODD HEAD SHAPE

Did your baby come out with a cone head? This is totally normal and should resolve itself with time. Babies have two soft spots on their skull called fontanelles. One is on the top of the head and one is at the back. These soft spots help the head to compress so the baby can easily pass through the birth canal. This process is called molding, and it can cause the baby's head to look a little misshapen. Keep these soft spots in mind as you and Mom cuddle with the baby and work on breastfeeding. For the first few weeks, you don't want to put much pressure on your baby's little noggin.

MEDICAL INTERVENTIONS

If you give birth in a hospital, there are a few standard interventions you should expect. It's good to know about these ahead of time so you can talk to your doctor or pediatrician if you have any questions.

Antibiotic cream will be dabbed in your baby's eyes. This preventative measure protects your baby's eyes from chlamydia, gonorrhea, or anything else that she might have been exposed to in the birth canal. Does Mom have any of these STDs? Probably not. However, many states require that your baby receives this cream. It causes a tiny bit of blurriness for the baby's eyes but no discomfort or lasting effects.

Vitamin K will be injected into your baby's leg to protect against vitamin K deficiency bleeding (VKDB). Less than 2 percent of babies are affected by this disorder (Zipursky 1999), but if your otherwise healthy-looking baby has this condition, her blood will be unable to clot and she could end up hemorrhaging. The good news is that one dose of vitamin K is all it takes to reduce the chances of VKDB significantly.

A vaccination is usually administered with the vitamin K shot to protect against hepatitis B. Both injections can be administered while the baby is lying on Mom's chest or nursing.

If you have questions or concerns about any of these medical interventions, definitely talk to your doc or pediatrician about your options prior to birth.

HOW BIG IS MY BABY?

You know you've been waiting to find out your baby's stats, Dad. At some point, a nurse will gently weigh your baby and measure his or her height and head circumference. This is a great opportunity to direct some applause in Mom's direction. Regardless of how big your baby is, she carried this little person in her body for quite a while, and she deserves a standing ovation!

SKIN-TO-SKIN CONTACT

In between the tasks that the nursing staff is conducting, you and Mom should get as much skin-to-skin contact with that little baby as possible. Unwrap the swaddle, unbutton your shirt, and cozy up with your baby. Mom in particular should make skin-to-skin contact a priority. It will have a calming effect on both her and the baby and will stabilize your baby's body temperature and blood sugar. It will also initiate the production of nineteen digestive enzymes in your baby and get breastfeeding off to an amazing start, which leads me to my next (*and favorite*) topic.

The Lowdown on Breastfeeding

You may look at the title of this section and think, *Okay, time to hand the book over to Mom. She's going to be doing the feeding, so she needs to know the scoop, right?* Well, yes and no. Yes, it is important that Mom understands the mechanisms of breastfeeding so that she is set up for success and doesn't get discouraged. But, it is equally important for you to be informed and educated on the subject. Mom and baby have never attempted this task before, and they can use as much encouragement, guidance, and love as you can possibly offer. If you go into the breastfeeding experience knowing the basics about functions, latches, and positions, Mom will feel like you are her wingman not only in birth, but in everything that comes after.

Samar contacted me a few days after his wife, Kiara, had given birth to a little girl. He explained that they were having breastfeeding difficulties and asked if I would be willing to provide a quick consultation. Although I frequently do these consultations over the phone, I decided to pop over to their house so I could meet the couple and their new little girl.

When I arrived at the house, I could tell that Kiara was skeptical. Understandably she looked tired, and her eyes said, *Who the hell is this dude who is going to tell me what to do with my breasts?* But after spending an hour with the couple, helping them work on latch and positioning, Kiara's face relaxed into a smile. She hugged me as I walked out the door. "I didn't want Samar to contact you. I didn't think that a man would be able to help me. But you've been super helpful, and I'm sorry that I doubted you."

I get this feedback a lot from moms and dads. At first, they are confused that a man could not only understand and help with breastfeeding issues but also be a certified lactation counselor. I explain to them that I see my gender as a plus, not a minus. I'm able to view the task of breastfeeding from the angle of a birth partner and a father. Because I've worked with hundreds of couples who are working to perfect their breastfeeding technique, I have become finely attuned to the mechanisms of breastfeeding and can really help Dad to step in and be a coach and supporter. Many lactation professionals give all of their attention to Mom and the baby. I include Dad in my coaching because I really believe that he is a crucial part of the breastfeeding puzzle.

My goal in the following sections is to transfer all of my expertise and knowledge about breastfeeding to you so that you can support Mom as she learns this new skill. We're going to cover the basics of how breastfeeding works, and I'll give you the full scoop on proper latch and positioning and teach you how to problem solve when you and Mom encounter challenges.

BREASTFEEDING BENEFITS

Before we talk about the how-tos, let's discuss why Mom would want to try breastfeeding? You've probably seen the ad campaigns with the slogan "breast is best." Well, it's true; there are *so* many benefits to breastfeeding. Let me list them off for you:

- *Health benefits for the baby:* Breast milk is like the ultimate vitamin and immunity booster for babies. It is custom-made and specifically designed to meet all of their nutritional and developmental needs. Babies who drink breast milk are less likely to catch colds, viruses, and pneumonia. Some researchers argue that they are also less likely to later develop chronic health conditions, such as diabetes and celiac disease. Finally, the risk of sudden infant death syndrome (SIDS) is greatly reduced in babies who are breastfed.

- *Health benefits for Mom:* Mom's physical health will also benefit. She will be less likely to fight osteoporosis, premenopausal breast cancer, and ovarian cancer later in life thanks to breastfeeding.

- *Mental health benefits for Mom:* Oxytocin, the feel-good hormone, needs to be released continually in order for breastfeeding to function properly. Breastfeeding has also been known to decrease inflammation in Mom, which can help with depression. And, believe it or not, breastfeeding mothers tend to get more sleep.

- *Recovery from the pregnancy:* The uterus of breastfeeding mothers contracts back to its prepregnancy size much more quickly thanks to all of the oxytocin that is released. Some mothers also find that they lose their pregnancy weight more easily. Mom burns up to four hundred calories a day when breastfeeding! For this reason, nursing mothers need to take in plenty of calories. They need to take in fuel to make fuel.

- *Custom-made supply:* Breast milk changes and evolves to meet the needs of your growing baby. It starts out as thick and golden colostrum and slowly becomes flowing, mature milk as the baby grows and changes. It is kind of magical in this respect.

- *Inexpensive and portable:* I'm stating the obvious here, but people often forget the financial benefits of breastfeeding. You don't need to order breast milk from Amazon, and Mom takes her milk supply everywhere she goes. From a budgetary and practicality standpoint, it doesn't get much better than that.

BREASTFEEDING MYTHS AND FEARS

So if breastfeeding is *so* good for Mom and the baby, why don't all moms try it and then stick with it? This answer is complicated. There are many reasons—cultural, personal, and medical—why moms opt out of breastfeeding or give up quickly. I am careful to not pass judgment on a couple's choice about how they want to feed their baby. However, I do try to dispel the most common myths that might discourage someone from trying.

Myth #1: I won't have enough milk. I feel like this myth has two origins. First of all, after World War II, breastfeeding simply went out of fashion. More women were entering the workforce and baby formula was widely marketed as a superior food source. During the mid-to-late-1900s, new mothers were given very little guidance on breastfeeding. In fact, many women were given medication or a shot that caused their breast milk to completely dry up. This led to the false belief that breastfeeding is a challenging task that most women are not designed for. Second, many people don't understand the stages of breast milk. For the first few days of a baby's life, Mom will not produce much milk at all, and this discourages some couples. If Mom's milk fails to come in, or if her milk supply is low, there are plenty of things you can do to address these issues. More on this later!

Myth #2: It will hurt. This myth drives me crazy. Breastfeeding really shouldn't hurt. If the baby is latching on to the breast correctly, Mom's nipples shouldn't be in a lot of pain. Cracking, bleeding, and excessive pain are usually signs that the baby's latch is not deep enough. I am going to teach you about proper latch later in this chapter.

Myth #3: Mom can't breastfeed with breast implants or if she had breast-reduction surgery. Cosmetic surgery has come a long way in the last few decades. Many surgeons are able to complete breast augmentation or reduction surgeries without severing the nerves surrounding the areola and the nipple. I encourage moms with implants to massage their breasts, from the back of the breast toward the nipple, in order to help move the milk forward. If Mom has had one of these procedures, tell her to not rule out breastfeeding just yet. There is a good chance that her milk production will be just fine.

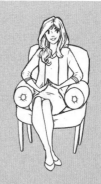

Counselor Corner: Fed Is Best. I think we all get the message that breastfeeding is incredibly beneficial for both the baby and Mom. For this reason, Brian makes it his mission to give moms and dads *all* of the tools they need to give it a good college try. Nevertheless, a limited number of mothers will not be able to produce enough milk to sustain their baby. Or they will be uncomfortable with the idea of breastfeeding for personal, cultural, or logistical reasons. *Yes*, we want moms to give breastfeeding a fighting chance, but let me emphasize that the most important thing is that your baby is fed and thriving. Brian was raised on baby formula. I was raised on formula. And we're doing just fine. Plus, formula has come a long way in the last fifty years! Companies have worked hard to make it as nutritious and wholesome as possible.

A 2015 research study found that women who planned to breastfeed and weren't able to (for various reasons) were twice as likely to suffer from depression compared to mothers who decided in advance to use formula (Borra, Iacovou, and Sevilla). For this reason, I encourage dads and birth partners to give moms plenty of reassurance, support, and love if bottle-feeding is necessary. We don't want to shame or judge moms if breastfeeding doesn't seem to be in the cards for them and their baby. Both Brian and I agree that as long as your baby is getting nourished, your little family is absolutely on the right track.

GEARING UP TO BREASTFEED

Although breast milk is an organic, naturally sourced food source that humans have consumed since the beginning of time, it is somewhat of a mystery to most people. I'm going to remove the myths and mystery and give you practical knowledge about the changes Mom's breasts undergo during pregnancy.

About halfway through Mom's pregnancy, her breasts begin to manufacture and store a thick starter milk called colostrum.

Around the same time, Mom might notice that her breasts are growing and becoming tender. Veins will become more visible beneath the skin. The areolas, which are the circles of skin surrounding the nipples, might grow darker in color and possibly grow in size. Mom might also notice small pimple-like bumps developing around the areolas. Tell Mom not to pick at them—they are there for a reason. Everything in Mom's body is gearing up to feed a newborn.

After the baby enters the picture, all of these changes to Mom's breasts begin to make sense. Newborn babies, left to their own devices, will use their legs' natural thrusting reflex to find their way to Mom's breast and begin sucking automatically. What draws babies to breasts? Well, let's start with those small bumps around Mom's areolas that I mentioned. These are called Montgomery tubercles, or Montgomery glands. They excrete small amounts of lubricant-like fluid that smells a lot like amniotic fluid and provides an oily barrier against infection. This fluid is familiar to babies because it smells like the liquid they have been living in and sipping from for months. It signals to them that they are in the right place.

Let's turn our attention to Mom's darkened, larger areolas and nipples. They act as a sort of bull's-eye for the baby, who can see twelve to eighteen inches away. Newborn babies will thrust their head and mouth at this target. The increased number of veins in Mom's breasts also have a purpose. They act as a natural heating and cooling system that can help to stabilize the baby's body temperature. Finally, as we discussed earlier, the skin-to-skin action has a calming and stabilizing effect on both Mom and the baby. Are you feeling as astonished as I am? Breastfeeding is amazing!

COLOSTRUM—THE FIRST STAGE

Let's talk more about colostrum. Until Mom's milk fully comes in, her breasts will produce small amounts of this thick, yellowish liquid. Some parents see this stuff immediately after the birth and think, *Oh, geez, breastfeeding is already getting off to a bad start. There's not nearly enough milk for our baby.* This couldn't be further from the truth. Mom will produce only teaspoons of this milk, but it is packed with nutrients. This stuff truly is liquid gold for a newborn. It has fat and is high in carbs, proteins, and antibodies. It also has a laxative effect, so it helps babies pass their first poop and rid themselves of bilirubin, a yellowish compound that is found in everyone's blood and poop. An excess of bilirubin can cause babies to look a little yellowish and possibly develop jaundice. Colostrum helps to flush out the yellow stuff.

Birth Guy Pointer: How Do I Know if My Baby Is Getting Enough Colostrum? I get this question a lot. You can't necessarily see how much milk your newborn is getting those first few days, and he might even lose a little weight, which is very normal. This can cause new parents to feel anxious and wonder if their baby is getting enough nourish- 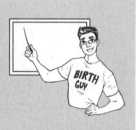 ment. Here's what you want to look for, folks: pee and poop. During the first twenty-four hours after the birth, you want to see at least one pee (one wet diaper) and one poop. While we're on the subject of poop, let me warn you that your baby's first few poops will look a little strange. They will consist of *meconium*, which is a black, sticky, and tar-like substance. Dad, this will be a great opportunity to step up and get the nurse to show you proper diaper-changing technique. The second twenty-four hours of your baby's life, you want to see two wet diapers and two poops. The third day, three pees and three poops. Easy formula, right? Your nurse will give you a chart to keep track of all the feedings and all of these diaper changes. If you're changing the right amount of diapers, your baby is getting plenty of milk. By the time you leave the hospital, you are going to be a pro at diaper changing and filling in charts!

Each feeding of colostrum will only equal about half a teaspoon per breast. When your baby is first born, their stomach is only about the size of the tip of your pinkie finger. Really small! These small amounts of liquid are the perfect size. The tiny drops of colostrum fall directly down the baby's digestive system and line the intestines with a layer of protection.

During those first few days of your baby's life, Mom will want to nurse eight to twelve times every twenty-four hours. This schedule will ensure that your baby is getting plenty of colostrum, and it will help Mom to establish a good milk supply.

TRANSITIONAL MILK—THE MIDDLE STAGE

Approximately three to five days after your baby is born, Mom's milk will "come in." Her breasts might grow in size and become firmer or even engorged. Yup, it might appear as if she had a boob job overnight, which she may or may not be pleased about. Mom might begin leaking more milk. This milk, referred to as transitional milk, is whiter and thinner in comparison to the thick, yellowish colostrum. It contains high levels of fat, lactose, and vitamins. Mom's milk is changing to meet the needs of your growing baby, and it is beautiful. Sometimes this change is a gradual one. Sometimes it comes on suddenly. Both Mom and the baby will need to adjust to this new flow and supply.

What helps Mom's milk to come in? For the most part, the timing is controlled by Mom's hormones. She needs to just wait and allow her body to do its thing. However, skin-to-skin contact and regular nursing sessions with your baby can definitely help to get things flowing. Throughout the baby's first year of life, Mom's breasts will know how much milk to make based on how much she is nursing. It is sort of a supply-and-demand equation. The more Mom breastfeeds, the more milk her body makes.

You may remember from the birth plan chapter that we listed some things to help with breastfeeding success in the hospital. If at all possible, you want to avoid bottles, formula, and even pacifiers for those first few days. While Mom and your baby are working on latch, and while you are waiting for Mom's milk supply to get stimulated, you want as much breastfeeding action happening as possible. The steady flow of milk from a bottle, or the supereasy suck of a pacifier, might set back the progress that Mom and your baby are making. The more breastfeeding that happens, and the more colostrum that is consumed, the more likely it is for Mom to establish a good milk supply after her milk has come in.

Waiting for milk to come in causes some parents anxiety, especially moms. I encourage dads to pull out their calming Jedi-like skills again in order to reassure Mom. You can let her know as soon as the baby is born that it is going to take about a week for her milk to come in. This will help her to relax and allow the milk to arrive in its own good time.

MATURE MILK—THE FINAL STAGE

About three weeks after your baby is born, Mom's milk will morph into its final form, mature milk. Ninety percent of this milk is water. The other ten percent comprises carbs, proteins, and fats. The milk consumed at the beginning of each feeding is the foremilk. It contains a lot of water, protein, and vitamins. The milk consumed toward the end of the feeding is the hind milk. It contains more of the fat necessary for weight gain. Because this milk comes toward the end of the feeding, we encourage Mom to fully drain her breast each time, so your baby gets the good fatty milk at the end.

How to Breastfeed

You're probably thinking, *Okay, I hear you that breastfeeding is good for the baby. I hear you that there are different stages of milk. But how does Mom actually DO breastfeeding?* This is a great question and ever so important to ask. Yes, breastfeeding is a natural activity that has been around FOREVER, but that doesn't mean that it will come naturally or easily for Mom and the baby. It helps so much to teach parents about proper technique and positions so that Mom doesn't have to figure it all out on her own. Just like when you play golf or strum a guitar, technique and positioning are everything. I'm going to break down the different steps and positions so that you feel like you have the full breastfeeding playbook in front of you.

IT'S ALL ABOUT THE LATCH

"Latch" is a word that you will hear a lot when it comes to breastfeeding. You'll hear it used as a verb ("The baby *latched* on to my breast without any problem.") and as a noun ("Let's see if we can get a good *latch* between Mom and baby during this feeding."). When I use the word, I am referring to how the baby's mouth and lips are attached, or locked, to Mom's breast. Latch is everything when it comes to breastfeeding success.

Many people believe that you just insert the tip of Mom's nipple into the baby's mouth and…presto! Breastfeeding commences. The truth is a little more complicated. Think about when you take a bite of an enormous cheeseburger. You squeeze the burger to flatten it out a little, open up your mouth as wide as possible, and thrust the burger in, trying not to get ketchup all over your lips. That's exactly what we want your baby to do. We want your baby's lips to look duck-like and to cover much of Mom's areola. We want the tip of Mom's nipple to go all the way back to the soft pallet of your baby's mouth. This will put less stress on Mom's nipple and help your baby to have a much deeper, effective suck.

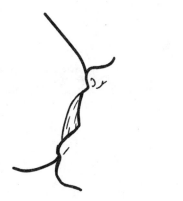
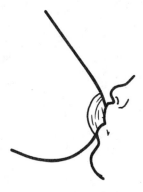

Deep Correct Latch   Shallow Latch

Not sure if you know the difference between the hard pallet and the soft pallet on the roof of your mouth? Here's a little exercise: Run the tip of your tongue along the roof of your mouth, from your upper teeth back toward your throat. You should feel a hard, solid surface that becomes softer right before you reach your throat. That, my friend, is the soft pallet, and that is where we want Mom's nipple to go in your baby's mouth. I promise you that your baby will not choke on Mom's breast. This deep, strong latch, with wide-open duck lips, will help your baby to get plenty of milk and will stimulate more milk production in Mom. It will also keep Mom's nipples from getting super tender and cracked.

Don't be surprised if Mom mentions that she feels some pain in her uterus or contractions when your baby is latched on properly. The deep sucking actually triggers a release of oxytocin in Mom and signals her uterus to contract. A good latch helps Mom's uterus to shrink down to its prepregnancy size. It's amazing how this all works together, right?

HOW TO ACHIEVE PROPER LATCH

After your baby is a few months old, he and Mom will be able to achieve a deep, solid latch without even giving it a second thought. But when the two of them are first figuring it out, following these steps might be helpful:

1. Gently squeeze the breast to flatten it a little and make it sandwich-like, keeping the fingers away from the areola.

2. Instead of aiming the nipple at the middle of your baby's mouth, aim it toward the nose and upper lip. Mom can even put a little bit of expressed colostrum on her nipple so your baby can smell the milk.

3. Gently tickle or tease the baby's upper lip with the nipple. This should trigger a reflex and cause the baby's mouth to open wide. Next, Mom should firmly insert her breast so that her nipple reaches back to the soft pallet. If your baby's mouth did not open up wide enough the first time, or if the baby's lips slip back down to the nipple, Mom should use her finger like a fish hook to break the seal and back her breast away. She should then tickle the baby's upper lip again, nipple to nose, which should trigger the wide-open mouth response.

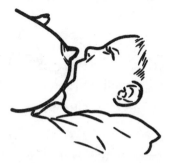

Align the nose to your nipple.

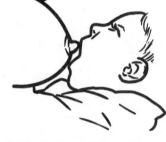

Tickle the baby's lips with your nipple.

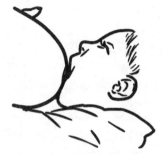

Wait for the wide mouth to latch on.

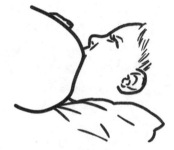

Lips are flanged, the chin is against the breast. A successful latch on.

Steps for achieving proper latch

How do you know if your baby is latching on correctly? Look for these indicators:

- Your baby's lips should be wide open. Both the upper and lower lips should be flanged out like those of a duck or fish. If your baby's lower lip is rolled in and you can't see the full lip, give it a gentle pull to help open it up.

- You should be able to see your baby's tongue when the bottom lip is pulled down.

- You should also see more of Mom's areola over the top of the mouth than the bottom. You want an asymmetrical latch.

- Your baby's ears should be wiggling and moving in a circular motion, and the jaw should also be moving in a circular motion instead of a rapid pistonlike motion.

- You don't want to hear clicking or smacking noises. Instead, you should hear a sucking and swallowing sound. During the colostrum stage, it should sound like *suck-suck-swallow, suck-suck-swallow*. After Mom's milk comes in, you will hear *suck-swallow, suck-swallow*. (If you're having a good laugh right now, I'm going to give you a pass. Let's move along, people. ☺)

- Your baby's chin should be touching Mom's breast.

- When your baby comes off Mom's breast, Mom's nipple should not be flattened or misshapen. We want the nipple to still look like a nipple, not like a pointed lipstick.

- Any discomfort that Mom is experiencing should end soon after the baby latches on. Superpainful breastfeeding is often a sign of a shallow, nipple-centered latch.

This might seem like a lot to keep track of, but it will all become second nature for Mom and your baby within a few weeks. If Mom can focus on getting a good latch early on, she and the baby will have more breastfeeding success in the long run.

FEEDING POSITIONS

Latch is not the only thing that is important when nursing. How Mom positions herself and holds the baby is just as key to successful breastfeeding. I usually encourage Mom to find a comfortable chair with great back support. A footstool or a small ottoman might help her to raise her feet a little and level out her lap. Many moms find that a nursing pillow is helpful. It helps to elevate and level out the baby, which will keep Mom from having to lean toward the baby or support the baby only with her arms. We want the baby's ear, shoulder, and hip to be in complete alignment. And, again, we want the baby's nose, not the mouth, aimed at Mom's nipple before the latch.

Making Mom comfortable is a top priority with breastfeeding positions. If she feels comfortable and Zen-like, the baby is more likely to feel comfortable, and breastfeeding will go more smoothly. You can help Mom by bringing her pillows, by helping her to adjust herself and the baby, and by bringing her drinks and snacks.

I teach new moms three different ways to hold their baby when they are breastfeeding. It might be useful for Mom to try each hold to find the one that feels the most comfortable. I'll start with the first position that I recommend.

Cross-cradle hold: For this hold, Mom should decide which breast she is going to feed from first. Then she should take the hand that is on that side of her body and use it to hold and support her breast. I call this the "boob hand." She should use the opposite arm and hand to hold and support the baby. We want Mom to gently support the baby's head around the neck, because the baby's head just got squeezed through the birth canal. Putting a lot of pressure on the head, or petting it, will not feel good to the baby and will distract her. I call this stimulating, or "stimming," the baby. We don't want to do that. Lastly, we want the baby's nose aimed at Mom's nipple so that they are both ready to try their first latch.

Football hold: Imagine a quarterback tucking the football under his arm as he dashes down the field. We're going for that same maneuver here. This position might be more comfortable for moms who had a C-section or have large breasts. Baby will lie along Mom's side under her arm, with Mom's hand supporting the back of the baby's neck. The baby's bottom should bump up against whatever Mom is sitting in, such as the back of a chair or a couch. Mom should be sure to bend the baby's legs at the hip so he doesn't push his feet against whatever Mom is leaning against. We want the baby to be comfy and focused on latching and feeding.

Side-lie hold: This lying-down position is restful, so many moms use it at nighttime. Both the baby and Mom lie on their sides, facing each other. Mom might have a pillow under her head and possibly one between her legs. It also helps to place a pillow behind the baby's back to keep her from rolling away. Mom can use the hand that is not under her body to adjust her breast. Although this is a great position, I usually encourage moms to start with one of the sitting positions so they can really see what is going on with the latch.

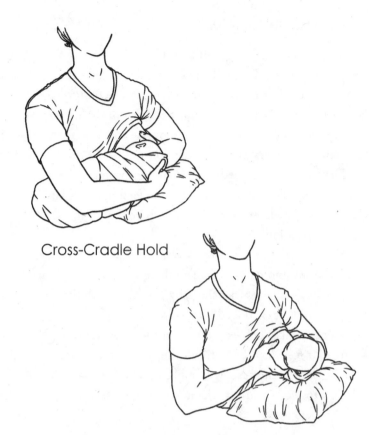

Cross-Cradle Hold

Football Hold

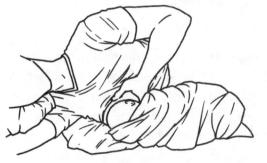

Side-Lie Hold

Three positions for breastfeeding

BREASTFEEDING DURATION AND SCHEDULE

The timing and length of breastfeeding sessions will change as your baby grows. The good news is that breastfed babies are usually pretty good at letting you know when they're hungry and at regulating their own intake. The first week, Mom should nurse eight to twelve times every twenty-four hours. That's a feeding session approximately every two to three hours. I know that seems like a lot, but the frequent feedings are going to nourish your newborn and help Mom's milk to come in. The feedings will last twenty to forty-five minutes, so Mom is going to be spending a lot of time in a nursing position!

Weeks two through six, Mom will feed at least every three hours. Many moms will feed with only one breast during each feeding. This ensures that the baby is getting both the foremilk and the hind milk at each feeding.

Occasionally, babies are excessively sleepy and don't wake up for regular feedings. Sometimes they can barely stay awake on the breast! If this is the case, you might have to occasionally wake your baby up to feed. You can tickle your baby's feet or side a little to keep him engaged.

HOW TO KNOW WHEN YOUR BABY IS HUNGRY

Babies use a universal language, called hunger cues, to indicate when they are ready for milk. The early cues are rapid eye movement and then waking up. Next, babies will begin smacking or licking their lips, opening and closing their mouth, or sucking on their hand or anything nearby. The active cue is rooting around on whomever is holding them. This might look like the baby turning her head and nestling it into your chest or the surface she's lying on, almost getting herself into a breastfeeding position. She might start squirming a lot and flailing her arms. The late cues are crying or moving the head frantically side to side. If at all possible, Mom wants to get her baby to her breast before the final cues kick in, so that her baby is completely calm and not "hangry" when attempting to latch on.

HOW TO SUPPORT MOM DURING BREASTFEEDING

Okay, so what do you do with all of this info? How do you best support Mom and your baby as they learn this amazing new task? Let's first take note of everything that is on Mom's plate: Her hormones and emotions are all over the place as her body recovers from the birth and ramps up for breastfeeding. She and the baby are learning a brand-new skill, which might not come easily at first. In addition, she is adjusting to interrupted sleep and a whole new way of being. For these reasons, you will play a major role in helping Mom navigate the early days of breastfeeding. Here are some ways for you to be the best breastfeeding partner you can be.

Pile on the praise, reassurance, and love. Tell Mom that she is beautiful and that you are so amazed and proud of her. Reassure her that it is going to take some time to feel like she and the baby have the hang of this thing, but that she is doing great. Remind her that her transitional milk won't come in for about a week. Cheer her on and tell her how much you love her when she is feeling discouraged.

Bring her water, pillows, magazines, her phone, or the remote control. When Mom is breastfeeding, she will have to stay seated in one position. When she gets a good latch, she shouldn't go anywhere until the feeding is done! Let her know that you are ready to be her server. Give her a little bell, if you'd like.

Help her get adjusted. While Mom and the baby are trying out positions, provide her with pillows and a footstool. As you would do with a new bicycle, keep making adjustments until Mom feels just right.

Keep the food and drink flowing. Mom will need to drink plenty of fluids to keep herself hydrated and her body cleansed, so make sure she always has a full glass of fresh water next to her. Not only will she need to drink a ton of fluids, she will also need to eat plenty of food. She was superhungry during the pregnancy, and she'll be just as ravenous while breastfeeding. Order in food as requested, and keep a little snack basket full of high-protein goodies next to her favorite breastfeeding spot.

Take care of yourself, Dad! Since you are going to be Mom's right-hand breastfeeding assistant, it is essential that you also take care of yourself. Snooze, eat, and drink whenever you can so that you can stay healthy and strong for Mom and your baby.

Make gentle suggestions. I've given you a ton of information in this chapter. You'll be going into the breastfeeding experience a lot more informed than most dads and birth partners. If Mom seems open to suggestions or feedback, share with her some of the info you've picked up from this book. Be gentle with your delivery and patient if she is not ready to hear feedback or ideas.

Contact a lactation professional. Last but not least, please do not hesitate to reach out for help. Your hospital or birth center probably sent you home with a list of certified lactation professionals. You can also do an Internet search to find one in your area. Or you can contact me, the Birth Guy, through my website. If you or Mom has any concerns or questions about breastfeeding, there are experts who can help you. Please don't feel like you and Mom have to figure this all out on your own.

TROUBLESHOOTING COMMON BREASTFEEDING PROBLEMS

Before I wrap up this chapter, I want to share some of the most common breastfeeding problems that I hear from couples. This is just an abbreviated list, so as I emphasized in the last section, please reach out for personalized help if Mom and the baby are struggling to breastfeed.

Issue #1: Several days have passed and Mom and the baby are still having a hard time with the latch. Some moms have inverted or flat nipples that cause latching difficulties while the baby's mouth is still small. In these cases, Mom can try a product made by Avent called Niplette, which uses suction to "train" the nipples or make them extend out more. She can also try using a silicone nipple shield to create a more protruding shape for the baby to latch on to.

A small number of babies have tongue-tie, a condition in which a little band of tissue tethers the tongue to the bottom of the mouth, making it hard for them to latch on and achieve a deep suck. If you suspect your baby suffers from this, have your pediatrician or a lactation professional take a peek. There is a quick procedure that can "untether" your baby's tongue.

Issue #2: More than a week has passed since the baby was born and Mom's milk has not come in. First, I would ask Mom and Dad if they are supplementing with bottles and formula. If they are, Mom's body might be confused and think that it doesn't need to make more milk. The solution in this case might be to increase the number and length of breastfeeding sessions. If Mom and Dad aren't supplementing, Mom might want to ask her doctor to check for residual placenta in her uterus. If any placenta is still hanging out, it might be releasing progesterone and keeping the milk from transitioning. There are also medications, herbs, and teas that are regularly used to increase milk supply. Encourage Mom to chat with her provider or a lactation professional.

Issue #3: Mom is complaining about excruciating pain as well as cracked and bleeding nipples. As I've said many times in this chapter, breastfeeding should not hurt. There might be an initial feeling of discomfort following the latch, but this discomfort should subside. Really painful nipples are usually a sign of a shallow latch. The baby's mouth is probably slipping down to the ends of the nipples, putting too much wear and tear on them. If this is the case, I would work with Mom and the baby to reestablish a good, deep latch. Mom should also try to wear loose cotton T-shirts that allow her nipples to breathe and avoid washing with soap, which might be drying her nipples out. There are also products available that can help to keep Mom's nipples moisturized, soothed, and protected.

Issue #4: Mom's breasts are engorged and painful, which is making it hard for the baby to latch on properly. After Mom's milk comes in, she might find that her breasts blow up like balloons and are painful. The solution to this is to release some milk, either through breastfeeding, hand expressing, or pumping. If the baby is having a hard time latching on to Mom's hard and turgid breasts, she can hand express or pump out some milk to soften her breasts and then let the baby do the rest of the draining. Occasionally, some moms will have a strong or forceful flow of milk that will cause their baby to back away from the breast or to not latch on properly. Again, the solution is to express a little milk so that the "let down" of milk does not overwhelm the baby. Mom can also try lying on her back and feeding the baby on top of her. In other words, she can use gravity to slow down her flow.

Issue #5: Forget feeding every three hours! Our baby wants to feed nonstop. When babies go through growth spurts, they might cluster feed, which means they might feed more frequently during certain times of the day. During these periods, it will be important for Mom to focus on good latch so her nipples don't get overworked or sore. It will also be important for you to support Mom more than ever since she might feel like all she is doing is breastfeeding. Keep the snacks, drinks, and love coming, Dad!

Issue #6: The baby was born ten days ago and still hasn't regained his or her birth weight. As I mentioned earlier, it is normal for babies to lose some weight the first few days after they are born. They should regain that weight and start to gain additional weight one to two weeks after birth. If your baby isn't getting bigger, your pediatrician will let you know during your newborn checkup. This could be caused by a variety of factors: proper latch hasn't been achieved, Mom's milk hasn't come in, or your baby is excessively sleepy and isn't eating enough. Talk to your pediatrician about your concerns and, again, do not hesitate to reach out to a lactation professional. Both providers are ready and able to help you with any breastfeeding concerns you might have.

The Magic of Breastfeeding

As you can tell from this chapter, I really do love the subject of breastfeeding. It thrills me to the core when I am able to see a family achieve a good latch and establish a healthy breastfeeding routine. If you and Mom give yourselves plenty of time and patience, there is a high probability that your baby will be a breastfed kiddo, and all of the amazing benefits will follow for your entire family.

BG FINAL SHOTS

✔ *Soon after birth, the hospital staff will need to complete some tasks with your new baby.* They will handle these tasks with tenderness and care, allowing you and Mom as much skin-to-skin contact as possible.

✔ *Although breastfeeding is a natural activity, it is helpful to read the owner's manual before proceeding.* There are so many magical and amazing intricacies that go into breastfeeding. Studying up on them will help you to be an informed and supportive partner.

✔ *Be patient and loving and reach out for help when needed.* Pile on the praise and support while Mom and the baby are learning this new skill. And remember, postpartum nurses, midwives, doulas, pediatricians, and lactation professionals (Like me!) are all willing and able to help you guys figure things out. There's no need to become a breastfeeding problem-solving expert all on your own.

CHAPTER 9

Bringing Baby Home

One January afternoon, I received a call from Hazel. I could hear the excitement and nervousness in her voice. She wanted to let me know that she and her husband, Connor, had been released from the hospital with their new little baby, Oliver. I had been with the couple four days earlier when Oliver was born via C-section, and I was stoked to hear that they were heading home with their healthy baby.

The next day, I dropped by for a postpartum check-in. The new little family was doing just great. I observed Hazel and Oliver during a feeding and helped Hazel to get more comfortable with the football breastfeeding position since her C-section incision was still healing. We worked on latch for a bit because Hazel was experiencing mild nipple pain and wasn't sure if Oliver was getting enough milk. While I was there, a friend dropped off a meal in a cooler on the front porch. In the back of the house, Connor's cousin was folding laundry. A fire was going in the fireplace, coffee-house music was softly playing through speakers, and Connor passed through the family room with fresh water and snacks for Hazel.

Does this idyllic postpartum scene sound a little too good to be true? I hear you on that. I'll tell you what Hazel and Connor did to set themselves up for success: they created a postpartum plan. They made a list of all of the individuals who could be helpful to them after the birth. They also planned out how they would make their home a soothing, relaxing environment and what they would do for self-care. Sure, there were days when Hazel was emotional and exhausted after an afternoon of cluster feeding. There were also days when the laundry and dirty dishes were overflowing and Connor and Hazel just shrugged their shoulders and sighed. Those days didn't happen as frequently as you might imagine, because the couple took the time to prepare themselves for the postpartum period.

In this brief chapter, I am going to share some hints with you about how to design your own postpartum plan and make the most of your first few weeks at home with your new baby. Before we do that, let's talk about putting together a nursery for your little one so that you come home to everything you need to be a prepared parent.

Making Your Home Ready for Baby

Most couples I work with like to set up a room, or nursery, designated for their baby. This is a place to put the changing table and all of the diapers. Usually it has a crib and a special glider or rocking chair for Mom to breastfeed in. As the baby grows, it can be a great place for the entire family to read books and hang out. When you're decorating, keep in mind that you might be spending a ton of time in this room, so make it cool!

I encourage couples to have the nursery set up one to two months before the due date. Mom can sit in it, play soothing music, and envision how she wants the birth to go. If you don't have an extra room in your house, don't freak out. Humans have been raising families for centuries without such dedicated spaces; even today, in parts of the world all family members sleep and eat in the same room. A nursery is a nice luxury but not a necessity. For families who end up cosleeping—that is, sharing the same bed—they might not use the nursery much at all. Once again, it is up to you and Mom to decide what is the best fit for your lifestyle. Regardless of whether you set up a nursery or not, you'll want to stock up on some supplies, which leads me to the next section.

LET'S TALK ABOUT STUFF

The truth is you really don't need a bunch of gear for a baby: Mom's breasts, some warm blankets, some diapers, and you're good to go. However, there are a ton of products designed to make your life easier with a baby—and they really do make life easier. Here's a quick list of baby items that you should consider stocking up on. Some of the items, as indicated, will not be needed directly after the birth but will come in handy later:

- *Baby clothes (sized from newborn to twelve months):* You can often fill up your drawers and closets with hand-me-downs from other new parents. Don't forget those cute little hats, socks, and booties.

- *Diapers (sized from newborn to size one):* Stock up on plenty of these. Let me warn you, Dad, you're going to be changing a ton of diapers. Don't forget a changing pad, baby wipes, diaper rash cream, and a diaper bin that closes really tight, for obvious reasons.

- *Baby carrier:* Wearing your baby is super popular these days, for both Mom and Dad. Babies likes to be warm and snuggly next to their parents' bodies, and parents get to walk around and get things done. Win, win! Baby-wearing advocates posit that it helps the baby to bond with Mom and Dad and to feel safe. When it comes to strapping a baby on you, there are several methods and brands to choose from. Ask your friends for their favorites or go to a local baby-wearing organization's meet-up to do some research of your own.

- *Stroller:* You know you can't wait to push that kiddo all over town. You'll most likely choose a stroller that goes with your car seat, which leads me to the next item...

- *Car seat:* You'll need one of these to take your baby home from the hospital or birth center. Make sure the one you choose is up to code and properly installed. (It might take a little work the first time you install it, but I promise you'll become a pro.)

- *Breastfeeding and bottle-feeding stuff:* A nursing pillow, a nursing shawl or cover, a breast pump, bottles, and a bottlebrush come in handy for feeding. It is also a good idea to get some nipple spray or cream for those early days of breastfeeding. Most hospitals will send you home with some baby formula in case there are breast-feeding difficulties, but I encourage you to consult with a lactation professional before using it.

- *Sleeping and cuddling stuff:* A bassinet, a crib, sheets, wearable blankets, and swaddling blankets can make cuddling and sleeping more pleasant.

- *Bathing:* Yup, there is a whole bathing industry for babies. You can buy a baby bath, baby shampoo, baby towels, and baby washcloths.

- *Feeding stuff:* You won't need a high chair or a booster seat (or both), bowls, baby spoons, baby food, sippy cups, and bibs for four to six months, so don't stress if you don't have them at the birth.

- *Soothing and entertaining stuff:* You know how you soothe yourself with your favorite music or that mind-less game on your phone? Well, your baby's gonna need some soothing as well, so you might want to pick up pacifiers, a baby swing, white-noise machines, a bouncy seat, and toys.

- *Safety stuff:* The only thing you'll need for the first eight or so months is a baby monitor, but after your baby starts moving and grooving, it will be time to babyproof your home with safety gates, outlet covers, cupboard latches, and toilet seat latches.

- *Health and grooming stuff:* To keep your baby clean, healthy, and looking good, you might want to pick up a baby thermometer, a bulb syringe, teething toys, a baby hairbrush, a baby nail trimmer, and baby-friendly laundry detergent.

Are you feeling a little panicky, Dad? That list seems pretty lengthy...and pricey. Here's the scoop. As I said before, a lot of the items above are not absolutely necessary. Plus, you will get most of this stuff from baby showers and friends and neighbors who are dying to get rid of all of their baby gear. Don't feel overwhelmed. You'll get the supplies you need, one way or another, and you can always make a run to the store if you discover you need something. (If you'd like to print out a checklist of what we just discussed, visit http://www.newharbinger.com/41597 and download "Birth Guy's Checklist of Basic Baby Supplies to Gather During the Third Trimester.")

Creating Your Postpartum Plan

So many of the couples I work with want to spend a ton of time discussing their birth plan. I tell them that birth planning is great... and important! I also remind them that the actual birth experience is only going to last a few days. For this reason, it is equally important to create a plan for how they are going to proceed *after* the baby is born.

In my experience, couples who go to the effort to make a thorough postpartum plan, with active input from Dad, have a much easier time coping after they've brought their baby home. Here are some of the things to think about when you and Mom create your own postpartum plan.

Help from family and friends: Many moms and dads are eager to have people stay at their house and help out after the birth. Others are more hesitant about this, especially if they are more introverted.

Sit down and talk to each other about what kind of help you would like after your baby arrives. Is there a relative or two whom you would like to invite to stay for a while? Does Mom have a best friend who can swoop in and help with chores and baby holding? Make a list of helpful and nonstressful folks who you can line up to visit or stay after the birth. And then be very direct and specific about how they can help you.

Meal delivery: Would it be helpful to have friends bring in food and meals while you and Mom are focusing on resting and caring for your baby? There are amazing meal-calendar apps that a pal can use to set up a meal-delivery schedule with family and friends. Be specific about what kinds of meals you want and if there are any allergies people should be aware of. If you would prefer to keep visits to a minimum, you can specify this on the meal calendar. Or, better yet, place a large cooler on the porch. Your friends can drop off the food in the cooler and come back for a visit when Mom and the baby are more settled. You might also keep handy a list of take-out food options and freeze meals in advance.

Breastfeeding and baby-care support: You and Mom aren't exactly sure how things will go after your baby is born. Hopefully, there won't be any big challenges. But, as I always say, it doesn't hurt to be prepared, right? Put together a list of lactation professionals and infant-sleep experts in your area. You can ask your health care provider or a local parent's group for recommendations. A postpartum doula can also be a wonderful resource. Doulas can come in and help with baby care and light housework, but their main focus will be supporting Mom in any way they can. Finally, make a list of parent friends who have had positive experiences with breastfeeding and baby care. They will love it if you call on them for encouragement and advice.

Older-sibling care: Will there be big brothers or sisters in the house? I recommend that you make an entire postpartum plan for them. Who will watch them during the birth and hospital stay?

Are there friends they can have play-dates with? Can relatives provide little outings to make them feel special? Prepare a basket full of toys and books that siblings can play with while Mom is breastfeeding.

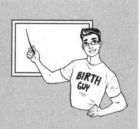

Birth Guy Pointer: Let's Talk About Sex. Quite frequently, when I am encouraging my clients to make time for their relationship after a birth, I get this question: So, when can we have sex? Great question, right? The answer varies from couple to couple. A Mom who had a vaginal delivery with no complications will usually be advised to wait four to six weeks after the birth to have intercourse. Moms who have had a C-section or other birth complications (such as a fourth-degree tear) might be advised to wait six weeks or longer. Of course, we also want Mom to feel ready both physically *and* emotionally. I encourage dads to avoid pressuring Mom to have sex while she is healing from the birth. This doesn't mean you can't find other ways to connect with each other during this time of recovery. Be creative in your efforts to maintain intimacy and closeness, Dad. Intimacy comes in many forms, right?

Self-care and relationship care: Last but absolutely not least, think about how you and Mom are going to care for yourselves and your relationship. Stock the house with your favorite magazines, foods, drinks, music, and movies. Think about times and days when you can give each other breathers and extra sleeping time. Make time for exercise, even if it is just going for a walk. Line up a cleaning service if it would be helpful. Look into new parents' support groups in your area. Start thinking about whom you would trust to babysit so that you and Mom can get out on the occasional date. Give each other plenty of praise, patience, and love. And, of course, reach out to a counselor or another professional if either of you feels like you are not coping.

You can download a copy of the "Birth Guy's Postpartum Plan" template at http://www.newharbinger.com/41597. Print out a couple of copies and fill them out when you and Mom are on a date, at least a month before the birth. You will be so pleased that you did after your baby is born.

Entering the Fourth Trimester

Many people refer to the first three months of a baby's life as the fourth trimester. Because babies are adjusting to the outside world, some believe that they would actually be quite happy to go back into the womb for a few more months. Let's think about it. Babies are used to a ton of ocean-like white noise in Mom's uterus. They're accustomed to darkness without a lot of light variation. They are also used to being gently bounced and swayed in the amniotic fluid as Mom walks and moves throughout her day. Finally, they are used to a constant flow of nutrients and fluids. Would you want to leave the soothing conditions of the womb? Hell, I wouldn't!

For these reasons, I encourage new parents to try to create a womb-like atmosphere for their newborn. Keep the lighting and voices somewhat low at first. A white-noise machine or a fan can create soothing and familiar background noise. Swaying and gently bouncing your baby on your body or in a swing can help calm them. Many people believe that swaddling babies tightly in a blanket or a baby carrier helps them feel like they are back in the tight quarters of the womb. Breastfeeding on demand is also going to help that sweet baby. And, yes, you knew I was going to say it, babies need as much soothing skin-to-skin contact as possible.

Your baby's days and nights might be mixed up at first, so you and Mom might be having a lot of nighttime action. For this reason, you will often hear people say that you should sleep when your baby is sleeping. I agree. Forget the housework. Forget the yard work. I usually encourage moms and dads to pretend that they are going back into a womb of sorts those first few weeks. Self-care, caring for each other, and tending to the baby are their number one priorities. The car washing and floor mopping can wait, I promise.

Counselor Corner: The Difference Between Baby Blues and Postpartum Depression. A new mother has a lot going on with her mind and body. Her hormones are shifting and spiking in order to help her recover from the birth and gear up for breastfeeding. Her sleep is disturbed, and her entire life is changed, as it is for you, Dad. For these reasons, it is very normal for a new mom to feel somewhat weepy and emotional directly after a birth. Commonly referred to as the "baby blues," these feelings of sadness usually show up a few 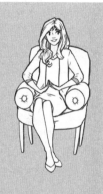 days after the birth and subside two to three weeks after the baby is born.

When the feelings of depression or anxiety do not go away, or if they get worse, Mom might be struggling with a perinatal mood and anxiety disorder. Current data show that at least one in seven new mothers experience some form of postpartum depression (Wisner et al. 2013). Here's the deal, Dad: You do not have to support or diagnose Mom on your own. If a few weeks have gone by and Mom is showing signs of depression, anxiety, obsessive-compulsive behavior, or even psychotic behavior—seeing or hearing voices, which only occurs in one out of every one thousand new mothers (WHO 2014)—*please* reach out for help. A doctor or a counselor can assess Mom and help her get the support she needs. The same goes for you, Dad. If you find yourself struggling with feelings of depression or anxiety weeks after the baby has been born, do not hesitate to reach out for assessment and support. There are doctors and counselors in your area who are ready to assist you.

A New Way of Being

When you come home from the hospital, you might feel like you have entered a new dimension. Everything looks, smells, and feels different. You might even carry yourself differently. You are a dad now, and you have so much to be proud of. Make sure that you allow yourself time to adjust to this new role. Consult with trusted friends or mentors when you feel like you're struggling. Lastly, trust your instincts, Dad. You will be amazed at your ability to rise to each occasion and be an incredible birth partner and parent.

Day by day and week by week, you'll gain confidence as a parent. As the years go by, you might look back at this time and barely remember holding your tiny little baby. Believe me, I've raised two of them, and they are big now! For this reason, make an effort to breathe it all in and appreciate every moment—even the late-night, baby-screaming, hall-pacing moments. Before you know it, you're going to be pushing your kid on a new bike instead of in a stroller, and it will feel like all of the work and struggle was truly worth it.

We've covered a ton of information in this book, my friend. Don't worry if you haven't absorbed all of it. You can pull the book out as needed and use it as a reference manual. Remind yourself that you're going into the birth experience with far more information and knowledge than most birth and parenting partners out there. You've got this thing. I have faith in you! Go forth and be the badass partner that you are!

Acknowledgments

Behind every great book is a slew of great people, and we certainly had a whole delivery room full of incredible individuals contributing to the birth of this book. Many thanks to Allison Cohen, our agent at Gersh, for believing so passionately in the Rocking Dads mission and for connecting us with the perfect publisher. Thanks to the many fine folks at New Harbinger Publications: Wendy Millstine, for falling in love with the proposal and getting us in the door. Jess O'Brien, for overseeing the gestation of our book while remaining cool and calm every step of the way. Caleb Beckwith, for masterfully shaping and editing our manuscript and throwing in ample encouragement when we were deep in labor. James Lainsbury, our copy editor, for your incredible attention to detail and focus on delivering a flawless finished product. Many thanks to everyone else at New Harbinger who worked so hard behind the scenes to shape the text and announce the birth of our book to the world: Julie Bennett, Karen Hathaway, Amy Shoup, Fiona Hannigan, Analis Souza, Jesse Burson, Michele Waters-Kermes, Lisa Gunther, Georgia Kolias, Jhoanna Valencia, and so many more. We wouldn't be book parents without you wonderful people!

Huge thanks to our illustrator, Isabel Hillock Davidson, for turning our words into pictures and making us look young and fabulous.

Thanks to Dr. Kelly Morales and lactation guru Lyra Smith-Hosford, for sharing your enthusiasm and expertise and for helping us produce an accurate and current guide.

From Brian: I have so many people to thank who have supported and inspired me on my Birth Guy journey: Eva and Daisy Salmon,

Chris Pegula, Joseph, Farrah and Noah Gonzalez, the BabyVision crew, Deanna Huerta, Kelly and Lando Morales, Sky Izaddoost, Clint Belew, Alex and Denae Schenker, Stuart Fischbein, Luis Moreno, Joan Corragio, John Caldarola, Ricardo Rico, Robbie Davis-Floyd, Desh Sharma, Craig See, Mark Bliss, Jason Murgo, Geri Collins, the labor and delivery staff at Methodist Hospital and the Women's Center in San Antonio, SAMMC labor and delivery, Sarah Davis, all of the fantastic physicians I work with and who have supported me, Robert Schorlemer, Bruce Landis, Heather Landis-Drexler, Michelle Fliehman, and all who have inspired me. Thank you to my uncle Bill Figueroa, who always gave me the confidence to reach my goals. I miss you here on earth. A special thank you to Kirsten Brunner, who joined me on this wonderful journey.

From Kirsten: Thank you to Cheryl Tyler for cocreating Baby Proofed Parents, and for urging me to carry on with the mission. Thank you to my entire family, my two boys, and especially my husband, Todd, for their unwavering support and enthusiasm. Finally, thank you to Brian, my coauthor, for taking me along on this amazing adventure of educating and empowering birth partners.

Birth Guy's Glossary

Active Labor. When Mom's cervix goes from five to six centimeters to seven to eight centimeters. This stage of labor usually lasts three to five hours, with contractions occurring every three to five minutes.

Amniotic Sac. The bag of fluids that surrounds babies, protecting and nurturing them in the womb.

Apgar Score. An assessment that provides a quick overall evaluation of a baby's well-being immediately after the birth.

Baby Blues. Feelings of sadness and weepiness that many moms experience soon after birth. These feelings usually subside two to three weeks after the birth.

Baby Brain. Fogginess or absentmindedness, possibly caused by sleep disturbance and a developing maternal instinct, that many moms report during the second and third trimesters.

Braxton Hicks Contractions. Painless and irregular contractions that begin during prelabor.

Breech Presentation. When the baby is positioned feet down (instead of head down) in the womb.

Cervix. The cylinder-shaped neck of tissue that connects the vagina and uterus, or womb.

Cesarean Section (C-Section). Surgery to remove a baby from the mother's abdomen.

Contractions. The periodic tightening and relaxing of the uterine muscle that helps the cervix to open up.

Chorioamnionitis. A bacterial infection that can occur in the amniotic sac, usually after Mom's water has broken.

Colostrum. The first breast milk. It is produced for the three to five days following the birth and is yellowish in color and packed with nutrients.

Dilation. The widening and opening of the cervix, measured in centimeters.

Doula. An individual who supports and coaches parents through pregnancy, childbirth, and breastfeeding.

Early Labor. The period of time from the onset of labor until the cervix dilates to five to six centimeters. This stage can begin weeks before the birth, or it might start eight hours before the birth.

Effaced. Describes the opening of the cervix when it has completely thinned out in preparation for birth.

Epidural Anesthesia. Medicine injected into the space around the spinal nerves in the lower back to numb the area above and below the point of injection.

Episiotomy. A small, infrequently used surgical incision made to the perineum, the muscular area between the vagina and the anus, just before delivery to enlarge the vaginal opening.

Fetal Heart-Rate Monitoring. Monitoring of the baby's heart rate during labor and delivery to check on his or her condition.

Fontanelles. Soft spots on the top and back of a newborn's head that help it pass easily through the birth canal.

Forceps. A birth tool that resembles large salad tongs and is used to gently pull a baby through the birth canal.

Gestational Diabetes. A temporary form of diabetes that a small percentage of moms are diagnosed with.

Group B Streptococcus. A form of bacterial infection found in some healthy adult women that requires treatment with antibiotics during the birth to reduce risk for the baby.

Hep-Lock (or Saline Lock). A small port placed in the hand that can be connected to an IV if needed but will allow Mom to have more mobility during labor.

Human Chorionic Gonadotropin (hCG). A hormone that shows up in Mom's body after fertilization has occurred.

Hyperemesis Gravidarum. Extreme morning sickness that can lead to hospitalization or IV hydration, or both.

Inducing Labor (or Labor Induction). The use of medical interventions to kick-start labor when it hasn't started on its own.

Intravenous Therapy (IV). The infusion of liquid substances directly into a vein, usually through a hand or an arm.

Latch. How the baby's mouth and lips are attached, or locked on to, the breast during breastfeeding.

Lightening. When the baby begins to "drop," or descend, lower in Mom's pelvis in preparation for birth.

Mature Milk. The final stage of breast milk that arrives approximately three weeks after the birth. It is mostly water with a smaller percentage of carbs, proteins, and fats.

Mucus Plug. A gooey, gelatinous plug that blocks the cervical canal and protects the uterus from bacteria and pathogens and might fall out during prelabor or early labor.

Neonatal Intensive Care Unit (NICU). Where premature babies and seriously ill babies stay in the hospital while healing and growing.

Oligohydramnios. A relatively rare condition in which there is not enough fluid in the amniotic sac to protect and cushion the baby.

Perinatal Mood and Anxiety Disorders (PMAD). Depression, anxiety, or other mood disorders that Mom may experience before or after the birth.

Perineal Massage. A form of massage that can help relax, stretch, and open the vaginal opening and reduce tearing to the perineum during childbirth.

Pitocin. A synthetic form of oxytocin that is administered through an IV in order to induce labor or help Mom deliver the placenta.

Placenta. A flattened, circular organ that delivers nutrients and fluids to the baby through the umbilical cord during pregnancy.

Placenta Previa. A condition in which the placenta covers the cervix and blocks the baby's exit.

Precipitous Labor (or Rapid Labor). Really fast labor that lasts between three and five hours.

Preeclampsia. A medical condition characterized by high blood pressure, swelling of the hands and feet, and protein in the urine.

Prelabor. Changes to Mom's body that begin one to four weeks before labor begins, signaling that Mom's body is preparing for the birth.

Premature Birth. A birth that occurs before the pregnancy has reached thirty-seven weeks.

Rebozo Scarf. A long, colorful scarf that comes in handy during active labor.

Relaxin. A hormone that helps Mom's ligaments to loosen in preparation for the birth.

Spinal Block. The injection of medicine directly into the spinal fluid that causes numbness in the lower half of the body.

Sweeping (or Stripping) of Membranes. When the provider inserts a finger into Mom's vagina and manually separates the amniotic sac from the lower part of the uterus to induce labor.

Systemic Medications. Painkillers that affect the entire body, not just one area of it.

Transition. The stage of labor before pushing begins when the cervix dilates from eight to ten centimeters.

Transitional Milk. The second stage of breast milk (when the "milk comes in"), lasting from five days to three weeks postbirth.

Triage Room. Where moms are assessed and evaluated in the hospital to see how far along they are in labor.

Ultrasound Imaging. The use of sound waves to produce pictures of the inside of the body.

Umbilical Cord. A thick ropelike tube that connects the baby to the placenta and delivers all of the nutrients the baby needs during pregnancy.

Vacuum Extractor. A tool that gently pulls on the baby's head, using suction, when the baby is stuck in the birth canal.

Vernix. A white waxy coating that usually covers a baby after the birth.

References

ACOG (American College of Obstetricians and Gynecologists). 2009. "ACOG Practice Bulletin No. 107: Induction of Labor." *Obstetrics and Gynecology* 114: 386–397.

Acosta, J., and J. S. Prager. 2002. *The Worst Is Over: What to Say When Every Moment Counts*. San Diego, CA: Jodere Group.

Ananth, C. V., J. C. Smulian, and A. M. Vintzileos. 2003. "The Effect of Placenta Previa on Neonatal Mortality: A Population-Based Study in the United States, 1989 Through 1997." *American Journal of Obstetrics and Gynecology* 188: 1299–1304.

Borra, C., M. Iacovou, and A. Sevilla. 2015. "New Evidence on Breastfeeding and Postpartum Depression: The Importance of Understanding Women's Intentions." *Maternal and Child Health Journal* 18: 897–907.

Buhle, J., B. Stevens, J. Friedman and T. Wager. 2012 "Distraction and Placebo: Two Separate Routes to Pain Control." *Psychological Science* 23: 246-253.

Carroll, J. S., and W. J. Doherty. 2003. "Evaluating the Effectiveness of Premarital Prevention Programs: A Meta-Analytic Review of Outcome Research." *Family Relations* 52: 105–118.

Christensen, A., D. C. Atkins, B. Baucom, and J. Yi. 2010. "Marital Status and Satisfaction Five Years Following a Randomized Clinical Trial Comparing Traditional Versus Integrative Behavioral Couple Therapy." *Journal of Consulting and Clinical Psychology* 78: 225–235.

Cousens, S., H. Blencowe, C. Stanton, D. Chou, S. Ahmed, and L. Steinhardt et al. 2011. "National, Regional, and Worldwide Estimates of Stillbirth Rates in 2009 with Trends Since 1995: A Systematic Analysis." *Lancet* 377: 1319–1330.

DeSisto, C. L., S. Y. Kim, and A. J. Sharma. 2014. "Prevalence Estimates of Gestational Diabetes Mellitus in the United States, Pregnancy Risk Assessment Monitoring System (PRAMS), 2007–2010." *Preventing Chronic Disease* 11: 130–415.

Dietz, P. M., S. B. Williams, W. M. Callaghan, D. J. Bachman, E. P. Whitlock, and M. C. Hornbrook. 2007. "Clinically Identified Maternal Depression Before, During, and After Pregnancies Ending in Live Births." *American Journal of Psychiatry* 164: 1515–1520.

Edwards, M. S., and C. J. Baker. 2010. "Streptococcus agalactiae (Group B Streptococcus)." In *Principles and Practice of Infectious Diseases, vol. 2, 7th. ed.*, edited by G. L. Mandell, J. E. Bennett, and R. Dolin. Philadelphia: Elsevier.

Eskandar, O., and D. Shet. 2009. "Risk Factors for 3rd and 4th Degree Perineal Tear." *Journal of Obstetrics and Gynaecology* 29: 119–122.

Gabb, J., M. Klett-Davies, J. Fink, and M. Thomae. 2013. *Enduring Love? Couple Relationships in the 21st Century: Survey Findings Report*. Milton Keynes, UK: Open University Press. Available online at http://www.open.ac.uk/researchprojects/enduring love/files/enduringlove/file/ecms/web-content/Final -Enduring-Love-Survey-Report.pdf.

Gabbe, S. G., J. R. Niebyl, J. L. Simpson, M. B. Landon, H. L Galan, and E. R. M. Jauniaux, et al., eds. 2017. *Obstetrics: Normal and Problem Pregnancies, 7th ed*. Philadelphia: Elsevier.

Gottman, J. M., and N. Silver. 2000. *The Seven Principles for Making Marriage Work: A Practical Guide from the Country's Foremost Relationship Expert*. New York: Three Rivers Press.

Gruber, K. J., S. H. Cupito, and C. F. Dobson. 2013. "Impact of Doulas on Healthy Birth Outcomes." *Journal of Perinatal Education* 22: 49–58.

Harms, R. W. 2004. *Mayo Clinic Guide to a Healthy Pregnancy.* New York: HarperResource.

March of Dimes. 2013. "Oligohydramnios." Last reviewed June 2013. https://www.marchofdimes.org/complications /oligohydramnios.aspx.

Martin J. A., B. E. Hamilton, and M. J. K. Osterman. 2017. "Births in the United States, 2016." *NCHS Data Brief No. 287.* Hyattsville, MD: National Center for Health Statistics. Available online at https://www.cdc.gov/nchs/data/databriefs /db287.pdf.

WHO (World Health Organization). 2011. *WHO Recommendations for Prevention and Treatment of Pre-eclampsia and Eclampsia.* Geneva: WHO.

WHO (World Health Organization). 2014. *Trends in Maternal Mortality: 1990 to 2013. Estimates by WHO, UNICEF, UNFPA, The World Bank and the United Nations Population Division.* Geneva: WHO.

Wilcox, A. J., C. R. Weinberg, J. F. O'Connor, D. D. Baird, J. P. Schlatterer, and R. E. Canfield, et al. 1988. "Incidence of Early Loss of Pregnancy." *New England Journal of Medicine* 319: 189–194.

Wisner, K. L., D. K. Y. Sit, M. C. McShea, D. M. Rizzo, R. A. Zoretich, and C. L. Hughes et al. 2013. "Onset Timing, Thoughts of Self-Harm, and Diagnoses in Postpartum Women with Screen-Positive Depression Findings." *JAMA Psychiatry* 70: 490–498.

Zipursky A. 1999. "Prevention of Vitamin K Deficiency Bleeding in Newborns." *British Journal of Haematology* 104: 430–437.

Brian W. Salmon, Doula, CLC, also known as Brian the Birth Guy, is a doula, certified lactation counselor, and prenatal imaging specialist. He created the *Rocking Dads* childbirth class for birth partners, and the *Facilitating Fearless Birth* class for couples. He has partnered with over 20,000 couples in his ultrasound clinics, birth classes, speaking engagements, and hospitals as a doula. He is based in San Antonio, TX.

Kirsten Brunner, MA, LPC, is a perinatal mental health and relationship expert with over twenty years of clinical experience. She cofounded the website and workshop series *Baby Proofed Parents*, which delivers sanity-saving and relationship-strengthening tools to expectant and new parents. She is based in Austin, TX.

Actor-turned-father-turned-designer **Chris Pegula** is creator of Diaper Dude, a high-profile line of hip gear for dads. He has since been featured on *Rachel Ray*, *Ellen*, *The Nate Berkus Show*, *E! News*, HGTV's *Gotta Have It!*, *The Oprah Winfrey Show*, and numerous other TV and radio spots.

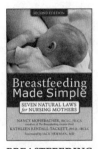
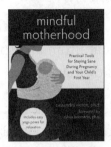
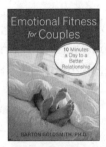
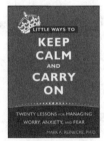
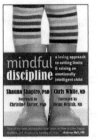
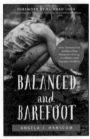
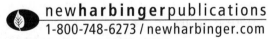

Register your **new harbinger** titles for additional benefits!

When you register your **new harbinger** title—purchased in any format, from any source—you get access to benefits like the following:

- Downloadable accessories like printable worksheets and extra content

- Instructional videos and audio files

- Information about updates, corrections, and new editions

Not every title has accessories, but we're adding new material all the time.

Access free accessories in 3 easy steps:

1. Sign in at NewHarbinger.com (or **register** to create an account).

2. Click on **register a book**. Search for your title and click the **register** button when it appears.

3. Click on the **book cover or title** to go to its details page. Click on **accessories** to view and access files.

That's all there is to it!

If you need help, visit:

NewHarbinger.com/accessories

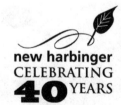

new harbinger
CELEBRATING
40 YEARS